Strong Medicine

STRONG
MEDICINE

George C. Halvorson

Random House New York

Library of Congress Cataloging-in-Publication Data
Halvorson, George C.
Strong medicine / by George C. Halvorson.
p.   cm.
ISBN 0-679-42980-8
1. Medical policy—United States.   2. Medical economics—United
States.   3. Insurance, Health—United States.   I. Title.
RA395.A3H345   1993
362.1'0973—dc20   93-28101

Manufactured in the United States of America
98765432
First Edition

This book is dedicated to my wife,
Mary Elizabeth Probst,
who took on a major extra burden over
these past several months so that I could write it.
Without her support and encouragement,
it would have been an impossible task.

I'd also like to dedicate it to my sons,
Michael, Charles, Seth, and J.D.,
who saw and heard a lot less of me during the writing process
than they or I would have liked.

I would like to thank Mary Lou Whaley for her help in putting the manuscript together, Maureen Peterson and Andrew Nelson for their help with the research, and the half dozen readers of my first drafts for making suggestions that clarified my points and improved the book immensely.

Contents

Strong Medicine

———————■———————

Chapter 1

FACING REALITY

It's time to face reality.

The health care delivery system and the health insurance system in this country do exactly what we pay them to do.

We pay them to create the most wasteful health care system in the world.

We reward our insurers for avoiding risk, increasing their administrative expenses, and serving as a dollar-skimming conduit between purchasers of coverage and providers of care.

As a result, we have the highest-cost, lowest-value health insurance system in the world, with the lowest percentage of people insured and the highest insurance-related administrative costs of any Western country.

At the same time, we pay our health care providers on a "fee-for-service" basis for procedures, not cures! There are thousands of billing codes in U.S. insurance for health care procedures; *there is not one single billing code for a cure.*

The sad truth is that we reward health care providers handsomely for complexity, redundancy, and waste, and we penalize them financially for cost-efficient care. And, because we are unique among the major nations in dealing with insurers and care providers as separate economic and social systems, rather than as two inextricably melded sides of the same coin, we have institutionalized a U.S. health care system in which the cost and value of care have become disconnected from one another in the decision-making process that affects almost all of our insured citizens.

To make matters worse, as the actual delivery of health care and the treatment of given conditions has become much more complex—often involving several caregivers in the care of a single patient—our organizational models for providing health care have basically been locked into the inefficient, splintered, nonsystem approaches of the 1940s—with a million of separate and fiercely independent caregiver profit centers competing with each other for their piece of the health care dollar at the expense of both efficiency and care quality.

The result is that we do not approach care on a systematic basis, with teams of providers focusing on the health care outcomes of a given population. Instead, we approach care as a series of unrelated events; our providers function with minimal teamwork and almost no sense of care continuity between care sites or even incidents of care.

A recent study of 185 consecutive comatose heart attack patients who had been brought by ambulance to a Rhode Island hospital illustrates my point.[1] The researchers—functioning independently of any regular hospital quality or utilization process—wanted to see what the survival rate was for those 185 patients.

What they discovered surprised them.

Every single one of those patients died. Not one survived to leave the hospital, despite the many thousands of dollars that were spent on their care.

The most important lesson from that example is not that all the patients died but, rather, that no one in the entire health care process knew that they had all died. When the researchers asked the actual caregivers to estimate how many of those patients had been revived and eventually sent home from the hospital alive, the caregivers estimated that a third or more had survived. These 185 consecutive deaths were invisible as far as the health care system was concerned. They were individually reported and then simply forgotten.

How could this happen?

Why wasn't there a payer—a buyer—somewhere in the process who said, "This is not an acceptable outcome. Let's improve the care process to get some survivors, or—if that can't be done—let's at least stop wasting hundreds of thousands of dollars on futile care for these patients until we figure out a way to save some of them"?

That would be a very logical question in any other industry.

Think about it. If Ford bought transmissions from someone and all of these transmissions failed, would Ford know? Would they respond in some way? The answer clearly is "yes" because that's simply good business judgment. In health care, however, buyers seldom use anything resembling that kind of good business judgment—for reasons that will be discussed later in the book. In fact, the buyers of health care coverage have, for the most part, blindly assigned their checkbooks to insurers, and the traditional insurance companies have very rarely gotten involved in tracking or even noticing any kind of health care outcomes for the populations they insure.

"Well," you might ask, "if there isn't any buyer or insurer tracking health care outcomes, isn't there some sort of outcomes-based tracking within the care system itself that could have identified the complete failure of the treatments being used?"

That's another very reasonable question.

The answer is, "No—we don't typically keep track of that kind of information in any systematic way."

For the most part, these types of tracking systems either don't exist in health care or are in their infancy. The reasons are economic, not medical. Providers of care are not paid for the outcomes of the care they deliver or for the additional expense necessary to track the outcomes of their care. Therefore, outcomes tend not to be tracked. (When they are, they are seldom reported.)

Instead, providers simply do what they are paid to do—and that is to provide "procedures."

Each of those 185 dead patients received lots of high-skill procedures in each of the independent profit centers in which he or she was treated: in the ambulance, in the emergency room, and—for those who survived long enough—in the intensive care unit. Each of those individual procedures was carefully recorded and included in a bill. These bills were probably carefully analyzed by the hospital's financial planning department to help determine if the care given to these patients was profitable. They were also probably studied by the hospital's market-research department to see if the hospital was continuing to maintain its target market share of heart patients brought in by ambulance. The ambulance companies and the many private-practice cardiologists involved in the care of those patients may also have studied the revenue flow that occurred and the profitability of their care.

But since no one was paying for outcomes, and since outcomes of the care given to those comatose heart attack victims did not affect either costs or revenues for any of the provider profit centers involved in the care, *there was no process in place for tracking the actual result of their care*—either as individual caregivers or as a "system" of caregivers.

Hard as it may be to believe, it took an almost serendipitous study performed by outside researchers to notice that all of the patients had died.

This is not an isolated example of how we take a nonsystems approach to care and to the results of that care. Think about it. Even though we now know how that hospital did in caring for these patients, we still do not know how the other hospitals in that town—or in your town—are doing with those same types of patients. Is a 100 percent fatality rate par for the course, or are there other hospitals and care systems that save 20, 30, or even 80 percent of these patients? If there are, what's being done to communicate these comparative findings to the public or even to the hospital in Rhode Island so that it can improve its care processes?

Health care outcomes can vary wildly from provider to provider.

We know from the brilliant pioneering work done by Dr. Walter McClure of the Center for Policy Studies[2] that the death rate for exactly the same conditions and procedures—carefully, fairly, and accurately adjusted for the sample size and for the relative severity of each patient's condition—varies significantly from hospital to hospital in the same community. In fact, the death rate in one hospital can be three times as high as the death rate in another nearby institution, yet these critically important results are unknown to the public and to the caregivers involved.

You can't tell which hospital achieves better outcomes by the prices they charge. According to McClure's "Buy Right" data, hospitals with higher death rates for a given condition are also, interestingly, often the more expensive institutions. In many cases, the lower-cost institution clearly provided better care, possibly reflecting better management for both care and administrative functions within that hospital.

Think about it. Heart surgery is a common event. We do 368,000 heart bypasses each year in this country.[3] Do you know what the CABG (coronary artery bypass graft) survival rate is at each of the hospitals in your area? Do you know that the mortality rate can vary by more than 100 percent between local hospitals? Would you like to know which local hospital has the better outcomes rate if you're considering heart surgery for yourself?

If you're reading this book, you're probably more informed about these issues than other people in your community. Even so, do you know what the early cancer-detection rate is at various clinics and physicians' offices in your area? Do you know that some clinics and care systems are four times better than others at detecting specific cancers before they get to the point where they are 90 percent fatal?

Do you know the preterm birthrate for the various obstetrics groups in your area? Do you know which care systems use screening programs and early intervention programs to cut the number of premature births by 50 percent or more?

Do you know what the cesarean (C-section) rates are for doctors in your area?

Ideally, in the highest-quality care settings, only 12 to 14 percent of births should be done by C-section. National averages, however, range closer to 22 to 24 percent, a number that is clearly driven in large part by the fact that U.S. doctors usually make about 50 percent more money per birth for performing C-sections.[4] C-section rates also vary wildly among provider groups. (There are even some with C-section rates approaching 40 percent—for no discernible medical reason.)

Unnecessary C-sections are poor-quality care. They involve major abdominal surgery and a slow and painful recovery time for the mother, and they are a terrible waste of our health care resources.

If you were a prospective parent, would you know what the C-section rate is in the clinic you would use?

That type of outcomes-based health care information is critical to the ability of patients to make good, value-based health care purchases. It is equally critical data if we want to start rewarding providers for improved outcomes, rather than continue to encourage high volumes of procedures regardless of their value.

Health outcome data typically isn't gathered, however, for four reasons:

1. No one pays for it.

2. The providers are afraid (sometimes with good cause) that the data will be misinterpreted, distorted, and used against them in some statistically or medically inappropriate way.

3. Comprehensive outcomes data is not always easy to gather, particularly since our current insurance systems are set up to pay claims, not to track outcomes of care.

4. Our health care providers typically function as independent-action units and profit centers, not as measurable, systems-based

care teams. Our health care approach doesn't lend itself to either statistically valid data or enforceable provider accountability.

More on that later.

If we want to evolve into a nation in which comparative health care outcomes data is considered to be as much a consumer's right as comparative octane ratings are for gasoline purchases, we need serious system reform. We must begin to treat health care delivery and financing as a unified system because, frankly, we can't fix just one piece of the problem.

BASIC FLAWS OF THE CURRENT APPROACH

Our current health care delivery and financing system has a number of serious structural flaws that need to be addressed both individually and as a package if we are going to reform health care in this country and avoid what could become a national system of bureaucratic rigidity and regimentation, regulatory gamesmanship, and rationing.

The basic structural flaws include

1. *Our current insurance system:* We now have a health insurance system that makes its money by avoiding risk, rather than by spreading risks across the broadest possible population and then working with health care providers in managing the risk to ensure both efficiency and quality. Instead, the current insurance world competes based on risk selection and risk avoidance, excluding from coverage many of the people who are in the highest need of insurance. Insurers compete today largely by using creative and skillful rating and underwriting practices that add absolutely no value to the delivery of health care or the ability of Americans to purchase insurance.

A more appropriate approach would be to have the insurers cover much broader cross sections of the population, with competition between insurers based on their ability to deliver high-quality, cost-efficient care, rather than their ability to avoid risk.

2. *Perverse fee-for-service incentives:* Total reliance on a fee-for-service payment approach for health care providers creates the equivalent of a sales incentive plan for unnecessarily complex and wasteful health care services. A more appropriate model would reward providers for the quality, outcomes, and efficiency of their care. That system would involve both outcomes reporting and prepayment for all necessary care for a fixed population of people. (This approach will be explained in more detail later.)

3. *Model T provider structures in the age of rockets:* Health care providers are operating as "solo practitioners" and individual profit centers in a profession whose science long ago mandated the use of caregiver teams. A far better organizational model would recognize that health care needs to be delivered by teams of providers in order to continuously improve both quality and efficiency and then pay these providers as teams, not individuals. The result of that approach would be vertically integrated care systems, involving doctors, hospitals, pharmacists, and other related caregivers practicing as a team to deliver consistent, state-of-the-art care. This would be a significant improvement over the current approach, in which each fiercely independent caregiver creates his or her own care approaches with no guarantee to the patient that those approaches will be either current, efficient, or outcomes-based.

Current estimates are that 20 to 30 percent of health care procedures done in this country are unnecessary. That waste will continue until providers can practice according to consistent and continuously improving care protocols and until they can be held accountable as teams for the outcomes of their care.

4. *Unaware purchasers:* Our buyers of health care coverage—including both private payers and the government—continue to purchase health care without demanding or rewarding either proven quality or logical, systems-based efficiency. Purchasers hold the greatest single influence and leverage power over the structure and

function of the U.S. health care delivery system—and, with a very few exceptions—they either do not understand their power or have chosen not to use it. Aware purchasers could restructure U.S. health care very quickly, once they understand the real issues.

5. *Silver bullet regulators:* Both at the state and federal levels, our lawmakers have a tendency to fixate on individual pieces of the health care problem and to attempt to solve, correct, or micromanage each piece of the problem without an understanding of the whole system or the potentially negative impact that their "silver bullet solution" will have on other problems. Our regulators and legislators do not take a "systems view" of health care reform, but rather a reactive approach that focuses only on select aspects of the problem.

Far preferable would be legislation that deals with the entire package of care delivery and financing issues and creates a solution by restructuring the care and financing system, rather than simply rearranging pieces of a nonsystem doomed to fail.

This book has been written to help people understand the significance of these issues and to offer integrated solutions. Subsequent chapters deal very directly with specific issues relating to physician practice, hospital incentives, perverse incentives created by current fee systems, the role of technology and technology manufacturers, the problems created by insurers and health maintenance organizations (HMOs), issues generated by the government and private employers as purchasers, and other problems created by lawmakers, rule-makers, and regulators. Chapter 7 deals with several current reform proposals and discusses the flaws and the strengths of each.

Chapter 8 presents some conclusions about how health care ought to be financed and delivered and offers suggestions about how we might make that type of system happen. (If you don't have time to finish the rest of the book, skip ahead to that chapter—but not quite yet.)

If this book contains information that is more practical and specific then theoretical, please consider the source. I write this book from the perspective of the front lines, not from academia. For the past twenty-four years, I've been involved in health care delivery and financing.

The health care organization I now serve as president generates more than $900 million in annual revenue. We own and operate two dozen full-capability medical and dental centers and contract for care with three dozen more.

Earlier in my career, I was involved in starting two HMOs from scratch and served as a senior executive for both a Blue Cross plan and a hospital system. I've directly and indirectly negotiated contracts and put together programs with hundreds of independent practitioners as well as with the best multispecialty medical practices in our region. I've worked with independent hospitals and hospital systems, and I've worked in joint ventures with two of the three largest insurers in the country.

I've sold coverage directly to consumers, to small groups, and to Fortune 500 companies. I've been directly involved in negotiating a number of government contracts and have helped implement a couple of state and federal pilot programs. I've served on three governmental commissions and a dozen committees and task forces whose role was to focus on health care cost and access issues. I've also been active in the national Blue Cross Association and the Group Health Association of America (the national association for HMOs.)

I mention this work experience to let you know that I am writing from direct experience about health care realities. This book is intended to give you a frank and practical insight into the way our health care delivery and financing system actually works and how it responds to the incentives that this country has created and continues to use. It might be controversial within the health care field, and some insurers and caregivers will probably find my focus on their financial incentives professionally insulting. That would be unfortunate, but that's a risk I'm willing to take because

I believe strongly that an informed public will make better decisions than a confused one, and we now have a public that is highly confused by health care issues.

Unless these issues are clearly understood, the likelihood is that health care reform in this country will focus on the wrong issues, and the result will be disastrous to us all.

CAREGIVERS AND INSURERS KNOW THESE ISSUES WELL

Although the perspectives this book offers are controversial, they are not unique to me. Far from it. The impacts of financial incentives on health care are known and discussed regularly by health care executives but rarely in public settings. Every health care business consultant knows these issues inside out, and many of those consultants could have written books on the topic that would make this one look pretty tame.

The public's ignorance on these issues is understandable, however, because those perspectives do not reflect the official image of either the caregivers or the insurers. I've given a number of speeches and talks—as well as offered some legislative and congressional testimony—on this topic. Invariably, the official public response of both insurers and caregivers is that I have unfairly attacked their professionalism, their motives, and their performance. But with amazing consistency, many of these same insurers and caregivers will privately admit later that what I described is also their view of reality and is, in fact, the way the system really works.

The truth is that the "incentive problems" that are discussed in some detail in this book are a dirty little secret known by just about everyone who practices and thinks about either insurance or health care, but they are not well known or understood (at least not as an interlocking series of problems) by either the public or by most governmental policymakers.

It is time for those issues to be made public.

Frankly, I don't believe that anyone can understand the

strengths and weaknesses of any health care reform proposal without understanding the points made in these chapters. My goal has been to explain each major point with enough specific examples so that you will be able to withstand the counterattacks that will come from the vested interests whose oxen are, I hope, well gored by this book. That means that some chapters will require careful reading. If any of them get tedious—or if the point is sufficiently clear—just skip ahead to the next chapter. Each covers a different topic, and each can stand alone to make its point. (If you're really pressed for time, just read the first five or six pages of each chapter. I suspect that you will find yourself reading additional pages in most chapters and will at least understand the key points of the remaining chapters.)

I hope you enjoy the book.

DOCTORS

A few months ago, in the physician's dining room of a local hospital, I overheard a doctor talking to a peer.

"I'm glad today is only Thursday," he said. "I've really come to dislike Fridays in our clinic."

"Why is that?" his friend asked.

"Well," the first doctor said, "a couple of months ago, my partners and I bought an X-ray machine for our office. On Fridays, we get together with the clinic manager and he goes through our charts to point out where we missed opportunities to take X-rays. I really dislike that lunch."

It was pretty clear that the clinic manager wasn't doing quality-care review on those charts. The goal of the meeting was to increase revenue, not to improve care. That focus on billable procedures by the clinic manager makes perfect sense, however, since we pay our physicians on a procedure basis and since clinic managers themselves are often paid based on a percentage of clinic profits.

A recent General Accounting Office (GAO) study showed that when physicians own laboratories, they tend to order .53 services per patient visit at a cost of $9.93 per service, while their peers who do not own labs order only .27 services per visit at an average cost of $8.68 per service.[1]

Coincidental?

Not very likely. The same GAO study showed that doctors who own imaging (X ray, magnetic resonance imaging, ultrasound) centers create an even greater cost impact. Although they didn't order more tests than nonowners, the average cost per imaging service in physician-owned centers was $96.51, while the nonowner physicians created an imaging charge per visit of only $52.92.

A *New England Journal of Medicine* article by B. J. Hillman, showed an even greater use of imaging when the physician made an in-house "self-referral" to equipment he or she owned. In the Hillman study, of more than six thousand physicians, the self-referring doctors were four times more likely to require a diagnostic imaging procedure, for the same exact symptoms, as a physician in the same specialty who had to make an external referral to get the imaging done.[2]

In addition, the average charge per imaging episode was 4.4 to 7.5 times more expensive when done by the self-referring doctor.

Dr. Hillman somewhat cautiously stated that "it is impossible to determine from our results whether the imaging practices of the self-referring physicians or those of the radiologist-referring physicians represent the more appropriate care. Nonetheless, the differences between the self-referring and radiologist-referring physician in the use of imaging are so large that some concern over the role of financial incentives must be invoked."

Another study, by Michigan Blue Cross and Blue Shield, showed a similar pattern: This study showed that when physicians own labs, they tend to order 6.23 procedures per patient visit and charge $44.82 per service, compared to 3.76 procedures per patient visit and charges averaging $25.48 per service for physicians who do not own their own labs. According to Charlotte Bartzack, the Blue Cross researcher who conducted the study, "There is no question that ownership interest leads to more testing."[3]

Interestingly—but not surprisingly—another recent study by the Health and Human Services (HHS) Office of the Inspector General (OIG) showed a similar pattern.[4] In the four years following the development of a new fee schedule for Medicare lab tests, the volume jumped 28 percent. The OIG also found that patients of physicians who own or invest in labs get 45 percent more tests than other Medicare patients.

These studies shouldn't surprise anyone who has looked at the way we pay doctors for care. We pay based on the number of services they provide. If they provide more services, we pay them more. Whether or not these services provide any value to the patient is not a factor in the payment process.

The result is an economic environment for physicians that rewards volume of services, whether or not they are needed (or even useful.) The current system richly rewards fee-schedule and claims-reporting gamesmanship. And the current payment system also richly rewards providers who use technology, creating an ever-increasing focus on the most lucrative, high-tech services.

The current system does *not* reward cures, positive or improved health outcomes, or proactive care of patients designed to prevent future health problems. We don't pay for improved health status. What we buy is process, and—*as always happens in a market environment—we get exactly what we pay for.*

The rest of this chapter will explain how medical practices are organized and paid. It will also explain how those organizational and payment models can lead to billing fraud, unnecessary care, wasteful and inefficient care, unfair physician reimbursement approaches, and an almost complete lack of accountability on the part of physicians when it comes to either recording or reporting the actual outcomes of the procedures they sell to us all.

Some of the information may be somewhat mundane, but it helps to take a practical look at the problems that occur in the front lines of fee-for-service health care, where medicine is clearly a business as well as a calling.

I had an interesting conversation a while ago with the president of a Fortune 500 company. He and a couple of members of his staff were explaining to me that the health care delivery system clearly lacked good management skills. A staff member suggested that we could bring prices down if health care would just dip into the ranks of business executives and transfer some of their talent into health care.

My response was, "Gee, if you are such good businessmen and they are all so bad, why is it that their fingers are in your wallets?"

Assuming that I was joking, they laughed.

"Think about it for a minute," I said. "If your section of the economy were growing faster than any other section—and if your profits and pay levels were at an all-time high—and if Wall Street was referring to major businesses in your industry as 'gold,' would you attribute that success to your lack of management skills? Would you attribute the growth to your lack of marketing skills?

"Health care is a business responding to a market," I told them. "It is very effectively absorbing every dollar you offer to it. If you think of health care business units as a bunch of fuzzy-headed, accidentally inefficient do-gooders who are immune from business pressures and incentives, and who are unknowingly absorbing your money, then you will never get their fingers out of your wallets."

I'd like to think that that conversation (and others that followed) were useful in helping one buyer see that U.S. health care is, in fact, a business and an economic system that responds wonderfully well to the perverse market incentives that the buyers in this country have inadvertently created for it. The problem is, we as a society have almost accidentally created incentives that reward a result we don't want and can't afford—a world of increasing costs and decreasing accountability.

The only way to create new and more appropriate behavior for the U.S. health system will be to restructure those market incentives and let the health world exercise its wonderful creativity in accomplishing new goals. In other words, if we, as a nation, want to purchase efficient, high-quality care, then we need to start explicitly paying for efficiency and quality, not for unaccountable volumes of independent units of service. Before dealing with the future, however, let's take a closer look at the payment and organizational approaches we use now.

I'd like to make it very clear that this is not an exercise in "doctor bashing." This chapter is simply about the incentives we place before U.S. physicians and their logical responses.

The overwhelming majority of doctors, I strongly believe, are ethical. The well-being of the patient is their first priority. Many fee-for-service doctors are relatively immune to the siren song of volume-generated cash. Others, while influenced by the potential for personal financial gain, do not knowingly perform any procedures or provide any treatments that would undermine a patient's health or reduce the likelihood of cure.

But when faced with two treatment alternatives for a given patient (one of which might create a $100 charge and the other with the potential to generate a $1,000 charge) and when both alternatives have an equal chance of working, the $900 revenue difference can be a persuasive tiebreaker for the physicians who will receive the money. That's basic economic reality as well as human nature.

In the interest of being fair to medical practitioners, I want to emphasize that the excessive imaging encounters and lab tests mentioned earlier in this chapter do not—except in relatively rare instances—present any potential danger or threat to the patient. But they do generate significant extra revenue for the physicians— and, therefore, additional cost for the purchaser of care. (The physicians involved would, I am sure, argue that the additional tests actually improve the quality of care delivered to their patients. They may even, if pressed, be able to identify instances where the additional tests were medically useful, and an objective medical review would probably agree in some cases. As the studies suggested, however, it's clearly not entirely coincidental that when questions of appropriate treatment arose, the care decisions seem to have been made fairly consistently in favor of the approaches that generated additional revenue for the physicians.)

The examples I've just given relate to physician investments in labs and imaging centers. That's not because those are the only areas where the reimbursement system may encourage excessive usage, but because they are among the most quantifiable areas of care. In actuality, tiebreaking between conservative and more lucrative and aggressive medicine goes on daily in doctors' offices across the country, and it occurs as often for very ordinary, primary-care issues as it does in high-tech, high unit-cost care.

"TROLLING FOR WARTS"

I asked a doctor who had spent years in private fee-for-service practice and then joined a large medical group where he was entirely salaried (and therefore no longer paid based on the volumes of procedures or units of care he delivered) what he saw as the major difference between the two practice modes.

"I don't have to 'troll for warts' anymore," he said.

"Troll for warts? What's that?"

"That's what my group called maximizing revenue from patients. In order to bring our billings and profits up, we looked at each patient to see what else we could do for them. If we saw a wart, we'd say, 'Just to be on the safe side, let's take that wart off.' The patients liked the attention, and the clinic partners liked the revenue.

"I found it demeaning, I'm glad that I don't have do it anymore."

It doesn't take an economic genius to see why trolling for warts makes basic economic sense in the context of fee-for-service reimbursement. The truth is that we don't pay our fee-for-service doctors to provide patients with overall improved health status. We pay them to do specific medical procedures (in an isolated context) for which we pay their piecework fees. If they do more services, we pay them more fees. And because some procedures are much more lucrative than other services, we clearly create an incentive to use the more lucrative approaches.

The fee-for-service system is basically flawed as a tool that cannot help achieve overall system goals of continuously improving care quality and efficiency because it doesn't reward or even recognize either quality or efficiency. In fact, it actively penalizes the caregiver who uses his or her talents to manage efficiently a patient's care since care management is not billable in fee-for-service medicine.

As an example, one health plan with which I am familiar has created a premature-birth prevention program that has reduced premature births to 47 percent of the state average. That program exists because the providers involved are at risk for the high cost of these births and are paid on a per-patient basis, not on a fee-for-service unit basis. Since they are prepaid for the total care needs of the patient, they can use their resources in the cause of efficiency and quality, and that's exactly what they did. They saved a lot of money—and improved the quality of care—by preventing preterm births through a special program. If these same doctors had been paid on a fee-for-service basis, however, they would literally have lost money by creating that type of program because there are no fees for the types of patient education, screening, and extra time for each prenatal visit for high-risk mothers that are needed to make the program work. As fee-for-service doctors, they would also have lost the fee revenue that comes from treating premature infants.

The difference in care that results from each of those two care systems is clear.

Some people defend fee-for-service payment approaches on the grounds that the fees accurately reflect the value of the services and the skill of the caregivers. It's even probably safe to say that most Americans believe that there is some rational relationship between the fee charged for a service and either the complexity of the service or the skill and training required to perform it. Far too often, this isn't true at all.

There is often little relationship between value and medical charges. Not only is the price attached to each service not based on whether or not it cures the patient, it isn't even related to the overall "value" of the procedure to the patient. Strangely, current medical fees are often not highly correlated with the amount of time or skill required to perform a procedure. Rather, specific fees for most services have been relatively arbitrarily assigned based on the initial price that the providers thought the market would bear when the procedure was first invented. In subsequent years, the price for a given procedure is usually based on how much price inflation the practitioners of that service have been able to coax out of the system in the time since the procedure was first invented. In many instances, procedures are refined and simplified over time, and the length of time and even the skill required to perform them shrink dramatically.

The fees, however, never shrink in the same ratio and actually usually continue to increase with inflation. In other words, as doctors learn to be more efficient in performing a procedure, the benefits of that efficiency accrue totally to them and are not passed on to the buyer. In fact, the reality is that the buyer usually pays considerably more per unit of physician's time for a given procedure as time goes on since the price goes up but the time spent on it goes down.

For one high-tech procedure—lithotripsy—a doctor recently told me that his total involvement now in that marvelous stone-dissolving process is to enter the room and "push a button." All other care is handled before he arrives by nurses and other technical staff involved. But his personal fee for the procedure has not diminished at all from the days when he had to be directly involved in the positioning of the apparatus.

Another perverse process occurs when the medical techniques for a given procedure do not become more efficient over time and the rate of increase in the fees for that procedure are relatively low. (That problem usually occurs when the procedure is done primarily on people who are under the Medicare or Medicaid program where fee increases are limited by the government.) When that happens, the physician cannot maintain his or her per-patient profitability by continuing to do the old procedure. In these instances, the physician has a clear financial incentive to maintain profitability levels by switching procedures for these same patients to something that pays better.

This means that another perverse result of the current fee-for-service payment approach is that perfectly workable and less expensive procedures are sometimes abandoned or avoided when the fees they generate are no longer profitable.

Switching to new higher-level procedures for a given condition often generates more money for the practitioner because, typically, new procedures are assigned higher fees than older procedures. This is true in part because the initial charge for a new procedure is not constrained by historical cost trends and because new procedures often are either time-consuming or require a currently scarce (and therefore very valuable) skill. This makes it easier for the physician to justify a higher fee level. As a result, the use of lucrative new procedures can spread like wildfire, even before any studies verify their efficacy.

Procedures involving scalpels, electronic cutting instruments, or any form of high technology also generate a lot more revenue than nontechnical diagnostic procedures or noninvasive medical treatments, such as prescribing medicines.

These payment imbalances and incentives are not lost on the physicians.

I have a friend who's a fee-for-service urologist with a large number of Medicaid patients. A while ago, I asked him how he managed to do well financially from such a heavily discounted payment source. (The fees paid by the Medicaid program tend to be very low compared to private-market fee schedules.)

"It's simple," he said. "We don't do many old procedures, just the new ones. The new ones pay okay, even for Medicaid."

He's a good man and an excellent doctor and I'm sure that the new procedures are best in a great many instances, but when they are only "as good" as the old procedures it's clear that dollars again influence the tie votes.

HOW PROVIDERS ARE ACTUALLY PAID

To understand how current reimbursement approaches directly affect physicians, it's important to understand the actual "business" of being a physician. The majority of doctors today still function as solo practitioners or in very small, single-specialty groups. Solo practitioners are small businesses in the purest form. They are paid on a piecework basis, and each procedure done for each patient generates a defined chunk of cash for the physician.

They hire their own staff, rent their own offices, purchase their own equipment, and bill their own patients. Money remaining after overhead expenses are paid belongs to the doctors, so they tend to know exactly how their practices function as businesses.

Private-practice solo physicians diagnose and treat their patients and then typically spend about six minutes per patient on paperwork. This results in a claim form that is sent to the patient's insurers, who, in turn, generate a payment to the physician. Those insurers can include Blue Cross and Blue Shield plans (the Blues), commercial insurers, HMOs, preferred provider organizations (PPOs), third-party Administrators (TPAs), as well as the government programs (Medicare and Medicaid). The solo-practice doctors also often spend evenings with their accountants, billing systems, and efficiency consultants to maintain their profitability levels.

Private-practice primary-care physicians in this country see about three to five patients per hour, depending on their specialty. High-volume practitioners sometimes see five to ten patients per hour.

Most of their cash flow comes from private insurers and the government and, increasingly, from HMOs or HMO-like entities. In almost all instances, these payers base their payments on the information that doctors submit to them about each patient.

To bill the payer, the physician selects one or more procedure codes from the fifty thousand codes listed in the *Physicians' Current Procedure Terminology* (CPT) code book for each incident of care for each patient treated. The CPT code and the doctor's standard charge for that service are then placed on a claim form (along with other data about the patient's diagnosis, age, address, employer, etc.) and the claim is sent to the insurer. Insurers, including Medicare and Medicaid, typically have a maximum payment amount assigned to each of those CPT codes. Insurers then pay the doctor up to that maximum amount without questioning either the validity of the charge or the appropriateness of the care, except in very extreme cases. (Most insurers will not pay for a hysterectomy on a male patient, for example.)

That *self-reported* fee-for-service billing approach clearly creates not only an incentive but an opportunity for physicians to increase both the volume of their services and the level of their billing with a minimal degree of outside oversight or review. In other words, the current system not only encourages volumes of services, it also richly rewards "billing gamesmanship." Most physicians do not act unethically in regard to billing practices, but, sadly, not all practitioners have resisted the temptation to make additional money by gaming the coding system. In fact, insurers believe that current health care cost increases have been driven, at least in part, by two recent fee-for-service billing gamesmanship trends called "code creep" and "unbundling."

Again, because the payment approach for care is both fee-based and self-reported, the system creates both perverse incentives and ample opportunities to create revenue by simply "fudging" the billing process.

CODE CREEP

Let me explain how code creep and fee unbundling work. These movements are important to understand in light of some current proposals to control health care costs by simply controlling the fees that providers charge.

As we have seen, the traditional health insurance system assigns a code to each care procedure and a price is assigned to each code.

However, because the same procedure can truly be more complicated if it is done on a person who suffers from multiple illnesses
or who has other conditions that make treatment difficult, the
usual insurance coding system takes into account the fact that the
complexity and severity of a given patient's conditions may war-
rant an increased fee. For example, a procedure that might be
relatively simple and brief for an otherwise healthy patient might
be more complex and time-consuming for another patient who
has diabetes, has recently had a stroke, or has some other com-
plicating condition or disease. The codes, therefore, appropriately
allow the doctor to report a given patient as a more complicated
case and, therefore, deserving of a higher payment. Some doctors,
however, abuse the system. For instance, a simple office visit (code
99214, with a $70 fee) might be arbitrarily upgraded by a doctor's
billing office to an "extended office visit" (code 99215 at $140), even
though the actual care given only justified the lower code. That
simple code change generates an additional $70 for the same work.
At a more complex level, a doctor doing a simple insertion of a
spine-fixation device (with a code of 22842-80 and a fee of $800)
might decide that there are mitigating factors that require an
assistant surgeon (with a code of 22802-80 and an additional fee of
$924), bringing the total bill to $1,724.[5]

Initially, those complex case codes were intended by the design-
ers of the coding system to be used in relatively few cases. The
definition of "normal" was intended to be fairly broad, and almost
all care was initially coded as normal. More recently, however,
doctors are finding a rapidly increasing number of patients whom
they believe justify the higher codes. (The doctors, I might note,
didn't have to figure this little billing game out on their own. An
ever-growing industry of "revenue enhancement" consultants are
available to help them modify their billing systems to look for
instances where "up-coding" can be claimed, justified, or at least
defended.)

Again, given the way we pay health care providers, some level
of code creep shouldn't be a surprise. One can argue that code

upgrading is probably inevitable to some degree, given the incentives and opportunities presented by the fee-for-service payment system. What business person, in any other industry, given a painless and unchallenged opportunity to redefine his or her product as having both a higher value and a higher price, could resist the opportunity to do so, particularly in an environment where the resultant price increases will not drive away customers?)

Most insurers now have computer programs tied to their claims-processing systems to look for cases of code creep. The process is hard to challenge in a great many cases, however, since medical judgment calls are involved and since the primary-source documents used to verify whether or not the upgrade was justified are typically the medical records that were written by the very same physicians suspected of doing the inappropriate up-coding. The administrative cost alone of challenging many of these cases is prohibitive for most insurers since the issues are complex and require involvement of at least an R.N. and possibly an M.D. to make the challenge successful.

FEE UNBUNDLING

Service or fee unbundling bears a significant resemblance to code creep. In an unbundling situation, a physician reports what used to be filed as a single procedure (with a single payment) as multiple procedures in order to increase revenue.

A simple example of unbundling might relate to the trolling-for-warts story mentioned earlier. As the coding systems were originally set up, a wart removal might be code 17110 (destruction by any method of flat [plane, juvenile] warts or molluscum contagiosum) and be worth $58. That $58 was intended to pay for both the office visit and the wart removal, and it was an all-inclusive charge.

Now, however, it is not uncommon for the physician to bill for the wart removal (code 17110) and then add an "evaluation and management" charge (code 99212) to the same bill. That additional charge adds another $35 to the bill, inflating the physician's income from that simple patient encounter by more than 60 percent.

Physicians who are particularly proficient at unbundling have also been known to add a "general supplies" charge (code 99070) to the bill to pay for such items as disposable equipment and towels used in the wart removal. That simple tactic can generate another $30 to $50 in revenue for the visit.

In other words, what once was considered to be a fair and all-inclusive charge of $58 for an in-office wart removal has become a total bill of $140 for some physicians.

As another example of unbundling, a physician can perform an eye exam and treatment on a new patient (code 92004, $58.50) and add an additional charge for a procedure that's normally part of the eye exam (determination of refractive state: code 92015, at $17.50). In this way, the physician can perform one procedure and create a bill for several procedures, thus turning a $58.50 visit into a $76 visit without adding any value in the process.

There are literally thousands of ways to unbundle codes.

It's difficult, at best, for the average claims examiner who has little or no education as a health care practitioner to identify these cases of fee unbundling. Claims examiners are trained to look for allowable procedures and then to price those procedures based on the insurance contract that the insured person purchased in order to pay the claim. It's darn hard for that examiner to look at a bill and say, "Dear me, I'm not sure that this case was complex enough to require an assistant surgeon." Some examiners, particularly those with nursing backgrounds, can do this, but it's a very difficult task.

As noted above, there are entrepreneurial companies whose function is to help clinics, physicians, and hospitals maximize their billing revenue by scouring the medical charts to look for opportunities to up-code and to identify opportunities to unbundle or bill for additional services. Computer programs exist to help them accomplish these goals. One company was quoted in *The Wall Street Journal* as saying that its "optimization" software can help providers legitimately increase revenue by 35 percent on Medicare bills.[6]

At the same time, as a defensive response by the insurers, other companies and computer programs exist whose purpose is to help insurers detect and prevent such code gaming. Most managed care companies have now implemented computer systems to help offset the uses of the code creep and the unbundling systems. The net value added to the health care delivered in this country by all of these expensive administrative games is zero. The net cost is significant.

Code creep and claims unbundling do no direct medical harm to patients, but they do generate expenses and inappropriately expend health care resources.

I mention these billing practices not to cast aspersions on the integrity of doctors in general or even on the doctors or other caregivers directly involved. Rather, I've written about those practices to point out again the perverse incentives that abound in the system we now use to purchase health care services. The overall payment system we have elected to use in our society creates both the incentives and the opportunity for code creep and unbundling and for selecting tests and procedures based, at least in part, on their revenue potential rather than their proven ability to improve health care outcomes. Again, we get what the system pays for.

INAPPROPRIATE FINANCIAL INCENTIVES CREATE OUR MAJOR COST PROBLEMS

It's important to realize that the problem of inappropriate financial incentives is central to the health care cost issue. It isn't a problem that can be resolved by simply fine-tuning payment levels, creating better billing rules, or even by seeking deep discounts on physician unit charges. Attempting to solve the problem of skyrocketing health care costs while retaining the context of fee-for-service payment as our primary method of physician reimbursement would be self-defeating and even counterproductive.

DEEP PHYSICIAN FEE DISCOUNTS

Some students of the health care cost problem believe that the solution to health care costs is to discount the fees paid to providers. For many reasons that are obvious to any experienced businessperson, however, the answer is clearly *not* to try to overcome the deficiencies inherent in fee-for-service payment by using discounts against these same fees. Discounting simply causes the provider of care to use other tactics to maintain revenue targets.

Think about the issue from the physician's perspective. When physicians who operate as small businesses with a fixed overhead that usually equals 50 to 60 percent of their revenues are asked to discount care on a per-procedure basis by 20 to 40 percent, it's clear that they have to do something to maintain their revenue stream.[7] Unbundling often seems to care providers to be a natural, logical, and even inevitable response to significant per-unit discounts.

Think about it. If an HMO, PPO, commercial insurer, or the government insists that you as a physician give them a 20 percent discount, and if your fixed office space, equipment, and support-staff overhead runs at 60 percent, then the discount will eliminate half of your take-home pay (since the 40 percent of revenue that isn't overhead is your personal income).

Deeper discounts make the situation even worse for you. If you are forced by market pressures to agree to a 40 percent discount, you, as a doctor and an independent businessperson, will have to spend *your entire discounted revenue simply to meet your 60 percent overhead,* with nothing left for your own take-home pay.

Discounts of that magnitude exist.

How is it possible, you might ask, for a care provider to survive in that environment, much less meet his or her personal income targets? We have seen that code creep and fee unbundling are two possible answers. Another frequently used approach is to shift the costs of these discounts to other payers by increasing the charges you use for all nondiscounted patients. Yet another answer is to increase the volume of services you provide to each patient while holding overhead constant (trolling for warts). Seeing additional patients per hour helps to increase hourly revenue with a minimal negative impact on your overhead expense. Performing more complex and expensive procedures (when a simpler approach would have worked just as well) is also a tactic that is used, as we have seen.

The easiest approach, however, may simply be to figure out ways to bill more per current patient while doing the same amount of work. The results are immediate and significant.

If, for example, after agreeing to a deep discount, you start doing a little code creep (to increase your revenue by perhaps 10 to 30 percent per patient visit) and you also unbundle a bit (moving your total, newly unbundled wart-removal fee from an all-inclusive $58 to an itemized $120, for example), then the discounts hurt a good bit less.

In fact, after agreeing to steep discounts, a doctor who unbundles, trolls for warts, and creeps the code could actually be making more money from a deeply discounted fee schedule—and that doesn't include the additional revenue the doctor can make if he or she also decides to increase the frequency of "callbacks" and repeat visits by patients.

PATIENT CALLBACKS

Callbacks are follow-up patient visits generated by the doctor to continue treatment, give test feedback, or simply "make sure the patient is cured." Callbacks may or may not be medically appropriate. In almost all instances, however, they are financially rewarding and they can nicely fill small spaces in a physician's schedule. A good example is sore throats. It's possible, and usually perfectly good medicine, to run a throat culture on a patient suspected of strep and then handle the lab test report by phone. It's also reasonable for the doctor simply to call a prescription in to a pharmacy if the culture is positive. These reasonable and highly efficient care approaches, however, generate no additional revenue for the physician beyond the initial office visit. The doctor who wants to generate additional revenue might instead tell the patient, "We've taken a culture and we'll call you if it's positive so you can come back in for treatment." The doctor then has the patient return for a very brief, but fully billable visit to pick up the same prescription that could have been handled by telephone. Or, the doctor who really wants to increase the revenue total might say, "The lab test will be back tomorrow. Let's schedule you for a follow-up visit then to look at the results and see what we should do next."

An automatic follow-up will generate another billable event for the doctor even if the patient doesn't have a strep infection, and, because the visit will be a very brief one, it will be especially lucrative. If the test shows the presence of strep, the doctor can take one minute to tell the patient, "You have strep throat. Here's a prescription. I'd like to see you for a follow-up in five days. Don't infect anyone else."

Or, if the test doesn't show strep, the doctor can take the same sixty seconds to tell the patient that he or she seems to have a virus and should drink lots of fluids, take aspirin, and call for a follow-up visit if his or her fever exceeds some level or if the virus hangs on more than "X" days.

In either case, that one-minute follow-up encounter can be coded as an office visit (code 99212) and the insurer can be billed for roughly $35 to $70 for a treatment step that could have been handled over the phone more efficiently.

As the lead doctor at one clinic recently told me when we discussed that very point, "I agree that a telephone call to give lab results can be both good medicine and a more efficient use of both my time and the patient's, but you won't see it done here. No one will pay me to make that phone call. I have to require the patient to return to my office to make any money."

The patients involved in this type of care, incidentally and very ironically, tend to like being asked to return for the follow-up visit, since they then feel they are getting an appropriate level of personal attention. Doctors who practice in this way tend to do very well in patient-satisfaction surveys, as well as financially. That approach has a very expensive negative impact on employers, however, since the patient has to take significant amounts of time away from work to travel to and from the clinic and wait in the doctor's lobby in order to get information that could have been given much more efficiently over the telephone.

The Canadian health system has recently experienced what appears to be a definite surge in callback medicine. Although the Canadian system is government-run with the government serving as the single payer, the primary-care part of the system is still based on fee-for-service reimbursement. The primary-care payment approach in Canada contains, therefore, the same perverse volume incentives we see in the United States. When Canada introduced a tight fee schedule in 1975, the result was an immediate increase in the number of services delivered. In fact, between 1971 and 1985, use of medical services jumped 68 percent in Canada.[8] Much of this increase was reflected in patients seen per hour of physician time, a logical result of the callback approach to revenue enhancement.

It also should be noted that the quality of care that results from unnecessary callbacks is actually somewhat *lower* than that from telephone contact. The patient who sees the doctor face-to-face to get test results usually has to spend time in a waiting room full of sick and contagious people and may not only acquire new germs but spread his or her own germs to fellow waiting-room occupants.

PHYSICIAN-OWNED EQUIPMENT MAY ALSO INCREASE REVENUES

As noted earlier, another way that medical groups and solo practitioners can enhance revenue is by owning and operating both lab and imaging equipment. Like most other medical developments, this trend has its merits and problems. In many cases, clinic-based

technology results in excellent and highly convenient care for
patients. In other cases, ownership of that technology leads not
only to overuse but to a poor quality of care since some smaller
practices cannot afford either the most modern equipment or the
highly trained technicians to run the equipment they buy. As an
example, a recent study by the Children's Hospital National Medical Center found that in some instances, small practices have had
poorly trained receptionists running lab tests with highly inconsistent results.[9] Some practices have unqualified employees taking
X-rays and even drawing blood or running lab machines.

These approaches increase clinic revenue, but often at the expense of good-quality medicine.

Again, the purpose of this explanation is to describe the incentive system we have created for our physicians, not to cast aspersions on their ethical behavior. I strongly believe that physicians
do nothing that they believe will harm a patient. The physicians
who choose to have their receptionists run their X-ray machines
probably all believe that the process is so simple that a fully
qualified X-ray technician isn't needed. In some cases, that may
be true. In other cases, it isn't. But in either case, the fee-for-service
payment system has created an incentive that can easily lead to
inappropriate provider behavior.

The Cost of Medical Education Creates Part of the Problem

It's important to remember that private-practice physicians in
the United States usually start their practices with a significant
amount of debt. Unlike other Western countries, where the government makes medical school much more affordable, becoming
a doctor in the United States is very expensive. The physicians
owe for medical school costs and, if they purchase a practice, they
owe for the practice purchase. They can easily start their practices
hundreds of thousands of dollars in debt. They have gone through
years of stress and misery to get through medical school, an in-
ternship, and a residency, and they, appropriately, feel entitled to

reap the rewards of the extremely difficult process they've been through.

I totally agree that physicians should be well paid since they do go through a rigorous and grueling educational process and they do society a great service. We need to continue to attract bright and capable people into the practice of medicine.

But in order to receive those rewards under our fee-for-service payment approach, solo practitioners too often need to function as hard-nosed businesspeople, and we ought not to be surprised if that sometimes results in revenue needs having an undue impact on care decisions. That is both human nature and economic reality.

We need a better way of paying physicians well that does not come encumbered with financial incentives to perform unnecessary services or deliver less than efficient care.

LARGER CLINICS

Physicians who join larger clinics and multispecialty groups ultimately face many of the same issues as the solo practitioners. Initially, those physicians tend to be hired by the medical groups at a comfortable and guaranteed salary level. It's fairly common, however, for that guaranteed salary to be replaced by a physician-specific production-based income after three to five years. In other words, after a few years, the physician's income depends directly on the volume of services that he or she can sell to his or her patients.

Physicians in those clinics who can't generate enough patient flow, procedure volume, and revenue to sustain their salary levels may take significant income cuts when the initial guarantees run out. They may even be asked to leave the medical group if they are perceived as poor revenue producers.

The incentive to produce encourages doctors to work hard, to be personable and service-oriented with patients, and to seek out opportunities to perform billable services.

Not all large groups use such financial incentives or pressure for their physicians. Some of the very best clinics in the country (the Mayo Clinic, for example) continue to pay their physicians a salary *throughout* their careers, rather than convert each doctor's compensation to a volume-based reward system at some point. That is one of the reasons for the extremely high quality of care at the Mayo Clinic. All medical decisions at Mayo are quality-based rather than revenue-based.

Multispecialty groups are even more likely than solo practitioners to own their own labs, imaging centers, and pharmacies. Frequently, they engage in joint business ventures with hospitals to run treatment and diagnostic programs that generate additional revenue for the clinics. (More on that issue in the next chapter.) They tend to be more sophisticated in their use of clinic management and billing practices and are less likely to be blatantly greedy in their procedure creep or unbundling practices since they usually have experts run their billing processes.

The role of multispecialty group practices will grow in importance throughout the 1990s while independent practitioners may well become obsolete by the turn of the century. This evolution in practice pattern is due, in part, to the increasing subspecialization of medicine.

Larger clinics are able to offer their physicians a better quality of life, easier call schedules than their "constantly on call" solo-practice peers, more benefits, increased economic stability, and better market leverage in their interactions with insurers and managed care organizations. The larger clinics typically also offer a better practice environment in terms of up-to-date equipment, technology, training, peer consultation, and support staff. The better-run large multispecialty groups can also offer the doctors a consolidated medical record that includes care given to a single patient by all doctors and all specialty departments within the clinic. This is a major quality improvement over the more disorganized individual practice environment, where each doctor who treats the patient keeps a separate medical record for that patient.

The multispecialty groups will probably also do much better in quantifiable quality of care comparisons once those comparisons become standard practice and will, therefore, be attractive to an increasing number of patients. Multispecialty groups can more easily standardize care along the lines of "best practices" and care protocols, and they can more easily provide systems-based care to patients.

Highly innovative, large, rural-based, multispecialty groups, like the Fargo clinic and the Dakota clinic in Fargo, North Dakota, may even help solve some of the major physician recruiting, support, and care-consistency problems that confront much of rural America. Based on their innovative "hub and spoke" network of rural clinics, they have the ability to place doctors on an as-needed basis in small towns without subjecting them to the rigors and drawbacks of small-town solo practice, such as no vacations, constant call, and no specialty colleagues.

The clinics of Fargo are now among the nation's finest because they have become truly regional medical programs—providing almost all care within a geographic circle roughly 150 miles in diameter—at a very high level of quality.

Multispecialty clinics, however, face problems of their own that result from the current reimbursement approach. Large clinics, for example, often run into significant internal battles over compensation that can result in the delivery of unnecessary care to their patients. The subspecialists within these clinics tend to be paid significantly more than their primary-care colleagues because insurance companies pay higher fees to subspecialists than to internists, pediatricians, and family practitioners. Primary-care doctors often resent these extreme payment differences and often argue that some portion of the fees paid to the specialists within their group should be shared with them since they are often the main source of referral patients to the specialists and thus deserve a cut of the specialists' revenue. Frequently, that argument prevails.

Again, the results of that approach are totally predictable. When the primary-care doctors in a multispecialty group are paid more money than their own fees generate in revenue, they, in effect, function as a "loss-leader" source of referral revenue for the more profitable specialties in their clinic. When they are, through that process, rewarded financially for the referral volume they create, then they have a clear incentive to make internal referrals. This approach guarantees a high volume of referrals (whether or not they are needed) and increased costs for all payers.

DISPROPORTIONATE FEES TO SPECIALISTS

The disproportionate fees paid to specialists are a problem in all areas of U.S. health care, not just large clinics. Those practices are simply reflecting the current payment bias of the fee-for-service fee schedules. These fee differences promote unnecessary use of specialty procedures and encourage a disproportionate number of medical students to enter into nonprimary-care specialties.

Recognizing the extreme and inappropriate variance in physician income among physician specialties, the federal government has been taking tentative steps to revamp its payment approach. Its aim is to have payments more accurately reflect the value of diagnosis and other currently underpaid primary-care procedures and to reduce financial rewards now given to procedure-focused specialists. The specialists are, of course, resisting this payment reform.

In 1988, a careful analysis of the relative value of various medical services was conducted by Hsaio and others.[10] That analysis resulted in a recommended revision of medical payment schedules. The modified process, called the resource based relative value scale (RBRVS), was originally expected to bring down specialist income by 30 percent or more. The Federal Health Care Financing Administration began in January of 1992 to use a modified version of the new payment schedule for Medicare, with the promise that as specialty incomes fell, primary-care incomes would increase by an offsetting amount.

But even as these promises were made, it was clear that the federal government, with its massive budget woes, would not be able to keep the entire bargain and resist the temptation to save money by simply reducing specialty payments while holding primary-care providers at the status quo.[11] It was even harder to imagine that the medical establishment lobby would allow those specialist incomes to drop to the degree proposed.[12] In one study, over half of the physicians surveyed began working with their hospital administrators well in advance of the RBRVS reform to try to recoup some of the income they were due to lose.[13] Although the outcome of the ultimately watered down implementation of the federal RBRVS system remains to be seen, it would be, at best, a partial solution to one portion of the cost problem. Since it continues to only fine-tune the current fee-for-service system, the likelihood of any significant long-term savings is very small.

A SHORTAGE OF PRIMARY-CARE PHYSICIANS

As you might expect from the large pay differences between the primary-care specialties and the procedure-oriented subspecialties, we are beginning to experience a shortage of primary-care doctors and a surplus of expensive subspecialists. Under a fee-for-service system with no relationship between the fees and the health care outcomes of the patients, this surplus of specialists will not create a competitive environment that will result in lower fees. In fact, since the subspecialists can, in effect, create their own market demand and revenue flow by determining which procedures their patients "need," the surplus in their specialties will not result in a market-imposed reduction in their pricing or in their numbers. Studies have shown that the specialist surplus will simply result in more marginally necessary services being provided at an additional cost for us all.

One study predicts that by the year 2000, the number of doctors per capita in the United States will increase by 22 percent from 1986 levels. Assuming that the doctors find a way to maintain their relative income levels, the increase in physicians alone could add $40 billion a year to U.S. medical bills,[14] and that number doesn't take into account the much greater expense that results from the hospital and other facility charges associated with each physician's practice.

As noted above, most of our new supply of doctors are aiming for practices in specialties in which the emphasis is on highly lucrative medical procedures, not on diagnosis-based primary-care specialties. Medical students can clearly see that the rewards for the procedure-oriented subspecialties are double or triple those of primary-care physicians. As a result, the vast majority of U.S. medical students now opt for nonprimary specialties. In Canada, 68 percent of the doctors function in primary-care specialties.[15] In Great Britain, 63 percent are in primary care.[16] In the United States, 36 percent of physicians are in primary care, and their numbers are falling precipitously.[17] Today, less than 20 percent of medical students are selecting primary-care practices.

This also is a natural result of our fee-for-service payment approach.

Given the way we reward doctors, this decrease isn't hard to understand. Income differences between specialties are great. A pediatrician's first annual paycheck after residency now runs at roughly $70,000 to $90,000 in a good market. An ophthalmologist, however, could start at $100,000 to $150,000, largely because ophthalmologists perform highly profitable cataract surgeries on an increasingly elderly population.[18] The pediatrician's income, over time, could range from $100,000 to $150,000 in a good practice, while the ophthalmologist's income could be double or even triple that amount. One might legitimately question whether these pay discrepancies accurately reflect the value provided by each specialty.

Pay scales like those of the pediatrician exist for other primary-care doctors, with base pay for family practitioners and general internists well under $100,000 in most markets. On the other hand, procedure-focused specialists like surgeons, obstetricians, neurologists, and urologists are all paid at ranges that approximate or exceed ophthalmology.

To add insult to injury, primary-care doctors are also finding their practices to be less interesting and challenging because, in many cases, the scope of their practice is narrowing. For example, malpractice insurance costs are forcing many family practitioners to stop delivering babies. General internists, once the referral physician for most heart patients, now find themselves referring most of their own heart patients to cardiologists. The primary-care physician is increasingly finding that he or she is serving more as a low-intensity-care generalist with a decreasing opportunity to treat more complex or more serious (and potentially more interesting and professionally rewarding) cases. These trends are much less evident in Canada and Great Britain, where the public gets better first-level care because there are many more primary-care doctors available to their patients.

PATIENTS DEMAND "SPECIALISTS"

Patients are partly the cause of this particular problem. Increasingly, the public wants to be treated by "specialists." In some markets, consumers are largely bypassing primary-care physicians to make their own self-referrals to specialists for relatively simple health problems because they assume that the specialist will provide a higher level of care.

The resulting practice patterns are very expensive and can be very wasteful. In a city like Boston, where there are very few family practitioners and the first line of patient contact is typically some type of more specialized physician, the cost of care significantly exceeds national averages and the level of care delivered for basic health conditions is often unnecessarily expensive.

The results of this environment are about what you would expect. A comprehensive study of hospital usage and costs in Massachusetts found that 1989 medical costs in that state were $1.75 billion greater than they would have been if medical charges had been equal to national averages.[19]

The study, conducted by the Boston University School of Public

Health's Access and Affordability Monitoring Project, concluded that $1.2 billion of the difference was "not justified by durably appropriate and legitimate explanations." The study concluded that the problem was due to "an elaborate, aggressive and costly culture of clinical practice [that] appears to have arisen in Massachusetts medicine, much of it seemingly centered in our tertiary hospitals."

PHYSICIANS AND HOSPITALS

The impact of physicians on hospitals is discussed in more detail in the next chapter, but it bears mention here that most medical subspecialists are largely based in hospitals and perform their most expensive procedures there. In towns and cities with more than one hospital, hospitals often compete indirectly for patients by competing directly for physicians since patients typically select physicians rather than hospitals and are admitted to the hospitals where their physicians practice. (As you will read in the next chapter, competition between hospitals usually results in increased costs to the patients.)

To compete for physicians, hospitals invest large sums of money in programs and equipment that enable physicians to perform lucrative (and often very worthwhile and valuable) procedures. Even though most hospitals are still nonprofit, in order to survive they need to invest money in technologies like laser surgery or magnetic resonance imaging (MRI) whose impact on the physicians' take-home pay is attractive enough to create physician loyalty to the hospital.

It needs to be said that many issues are involved when doctors decide which hospitals they will use, including convenience, culture, cooperation, and quality. A glance at almost any hospital's actual long-term strategic plan, however, will tell you that creating a practice environment that enhances the ability of the private doctors who use that hospital to make large sums of money is high on the list of factors that hospitals consider crucial to their success.

(That version of the plan is seldom if ever shown to the public or the medical staff, by the way.)

Hospital strategists count on the fact that the physician's decision about which hospital to use for his or her patients can be and are directly influenced by the physician's opportunity to maximize personal gain. Physicians, who often give "quality of care" as their top priority in selecting a hospital, might find many hospitals' perspective on their selection process very eye-opening. Hospitals tend to see physicians—not patients—as their customers. Patients are the revenue hospitals receive when they attract physicians.

In our current fee-for-service environment, in which hospitals and doctors are separate profit centers and are not held accountable as a team for the cost, efficiency, or quality of their combined care, that hospital perspective is not only logical, it's inevitable.

QUALITY OF CARE AND CARE OUTCOMES SHOULD BE MEASURED AND REPORTED

Interestingly, although physicians will usually list quality of care as their number one professional priority (and I believe they believe what they write), it's almost impossible to define or identify what quality care is. As noted earlier, medicine is largely unmeasured. Extreme examples of poor medicine are dealt with in our health care system, mostly through hospital screening processes mandated by Medicare or malpractice insurers, but there is almost no way to tell the mediocre practitioner from the excellent one, and there is no way for consumers to know which doctors, clinics, hospitals, or health systems consistently create the best results.

In fact, the fee-for-service patient/customer has almost no way of predicting, evaluating, or verifying the value of the services he or she is planning to buy. Even measurements as simple as mortality rate for a given condition are not typically kept in any usable form. Generally, outcomes-based care statistics are not available to the public, to the buyers, or even to other providers when they are recorded. This is particularly disconcerting when one considers that medical practice styles vary widely within communities and even more widely between communities.

C-SECTIONS ILLUSTRATE THE IMPACT OF FINANCIAL INCENTIVES ON CARE

Cesarean-section rates are a good example of this variance. In my home state of Minnesota, the Blues report that the C-section rate in some communities is as high as thirty-two C-sections per one hundred births. In other areas of the state, and in other practices, the C-section rate is closer to twelve per one hundred births.[20] The best medical researchers believe that a C-section rate of twelve to fifteen per one hundred births is more than sufficient to handle the medically indicated use of this procedure over a large population.[21] Any C-sections beyond that 12 percent number are, in the aggregate, suspect.

C-sections serve very well as an example of how we get what we pay for in health care because unnecessary use of C-sections seems to be almost entirely created by the way we pay for them. Because we pay doctors 50 to 100 percent more for doing C-sections, we get twice as many as we need. When we change the payment approach, the number of C-sections changes correspondingly.

The C-section data that is available clearly shows the impact of fee-for-service reimbursement on both costs and quality of care. Under most fee-for-service payment arrangements, doctors can charge insurance companies and patients significantly more money if they do a C-section rather than a normal delivery.[22] As a result, our C-section rate in this country has grown significantly (from 4.5 per one hundred births in 1965 to 16.5 in 1980 and again to twenty-five in 1988) and has to be looked at with some suspicion. This is particularly true in light of at least one recent study showing that "women with private health insurance are more likely to have a cesarean delivery than women with Medicaid coverage or no insurance."[23]

In Great Britain, where doctors are paid the same for a normal birth as for a C-section, the C-section rate was only 10.1 per one hundred births in 1983, compared to 20.3 C-sections per one hundred births in the United States in that year, and the mother-child outcomes in Great Britain are better than ours.[24]

Interestingly, numbers that are closer to the British results occur in this country in clinics where the doctors are salaried and do not make additional money by doing unnecessary C-sections. A few insurers have addressed this issue directly by reducing C-section fees to the level of normal deliveries. In areas and medical practices where the market share for the insurer was large enough for their payment decision to be noticed, I've been told that the C-section rates have dropped significantly.

REPEAT C-SECTIONS

The perverse impact of fee-for-service reimbursement on C-sections is even more pronounced for repeat C-sections than for first-time C-sections. Traditional medical wisdom used to be "Once a C-section, always a C-section," and mothers who had a C-section were told that all subsequent births would also be by C-section.[25]

This has proven to be both a false axiom and bad medicine. More recent studies have shown that 70 to 80 percent of women who have had one birth by C-section can and should have their next baby vaginally.[26]

The quality-of-care and quality-of-life impact on the mothers is significant when they can avoid subsequent C-sections. Instead of having major abdominal surgery, a long hospital stay, and a longer recovery period, the mothers who give birth normally have a one-to-three-day hospital stay and a very fast recovery.[27]

Why, then, are the actual VBAC (vaginal birth after C-section) rates in this country actually running closer to 10 percent than to the 70 percent number that is optimal?

The reasons, again, are *not* medical.

A California study of forty-five thousand women who had previously given birth by C-section noted that although close to 90 percent (89.1) of them did, in fact, have a second C-section, only 13 percent of those women had pregnancy symptoms that indicated that repeat C-sections were necessary.[28] Researchers further observed that the providers "with the greatest incentive to maximize reimbursement had the high repeat C-section rates."

The study further noted that only 4.9 percent of women with prior C-sections who gave birth in for-profit hospitals gave birth vaginally, compared to 8.2 percent in nonprofit hospitals, 19.8 percent in Kaiser Permanente hospitals, and 29.2 percent in University of California hospitals (with formal teaching programs focused on quality medical care). In Minnesota, where prepaid care is fully in place for a larger portion of the insured population, the percentage of women with prior C-sections giving birth normally in the best care systems now exceeds 50 percent, compared to only 15 percent in Minnesota's fee-for-service population.

This isn't just a cost issue. It's also clearly a quality of care issue, since C-section deliveries are associated with higher maternal morbidity and mortality than vaginal deliveries.[29]

VBACs are a reasonable and useful example of the impact of financial incentives on medical practice. Current practice patterns are clearly driven in some degree by the fear of malpractice suits, somewhat by the imposition of hospital-specific "community standard" peer pressures on physicians, and even somewhat by some uncertainty about the medical guidelines that should determine when repeat C-sections are called for.[30] But all of these factors need to be reviewed carefully in light of the clearly noncoincidental 400 percent difference in the VBAC rate between doctors whose personal income was directly affected by the decision to operate and those salaried physicians whose wallets were not fattened by performing the procedure. (Sadly, as the study indicates, even the non-fee-for-service physicians performed more C-sections than the retrospective reviews found medically necessary.)[31]

LET'S PAY FOR HEALTHY BABIES, NOT UNNECESSARY PROCEDURES

Ideally, medical providers should be paid for healthy mothers and healthy babies and the payment system should not encourage any particular medical procedure over any other unless that encouragement is based on clear quality-of-care standards.

Some private-practice doctors argue fiercely that the high C-section rate is driven by a desire to deliver quality care. However, if that were the case, the mere dissemination of clinical data to doctors explaining the medical appropriateness of VBAC's should cause them to change their practice to be in compliance with the best standards of medicine. The AMA, a generally conservative, pro-physician organization, has admitted that this education-based approach didn't work. According to a press release about C-sections issued by the AMA in February of 1990, "Dissemination of research findings, issuance of clinic guidelines by medical societies and expert consensus conferences generally have been ineffective. Those approaches have not altered practice patterns because they assume that decision making is guided solely by clinical factors."[32]

Obviously, those clinical decisions are influenced, at least in part, by financial factors, and the impact of fee-for-service incentives on VBAC frequency is extremely expensive, damaging to the patients, and counterproductive.

FEE-FOR-SERVICE PAYMENTS DO NOT REWARD QUALITY

To be fair to the fee-for-service doctors, a typical insurance company's fee schedule actually underpays doctors for the work necessary to accomplish a VBAC. Women who have had a prior C-section require slightly more predelivery care and education and need closer attention during delivery than do women who have not had C-sections. Most insurers' fee schedules do not recognize this additional effort and pay the same amount for a

VBAC as they do for a normal, first-time vaginal birth. That means that a doctor who expends the additional effort to accomplish a VBAC is relatively underpaid for his or her time. By comparison, if that same doctor simply elects to do a repeat C-section, rather than be underpaid, he or she can make 50 percent more money.

Fee-for-service fee schedules rarely reward efficiency for any procedure. Given the incentives we've created, the C-section numbers we see should not be surprising.

But is this type of problem unique to C-sections? Not at all. Anyone who is a student of the issue can recite numbers about the high percentages of medical procedures that are of doubtful value to the patient. As an example, more than 350,000 heart bypasses were done in the United States in 1990, and medical experts contend that up to 50 percent of them were "not clearly justi-fied."[33] (Again, the relationship between the high, possibly un-necessary volume of the procedure and the $300,000 average income for an "invasive" cardiologist is probably not entirely coincidental.)

The fees for these sometimes overutilized procedures tend to be high, and the specialists who perform them tend to be extremely well paid. They are well paid, however, only when they actually do the procedure.

They are paid less if they pursue a less invasive—but equally effective—nonsurgical treatment. It's hard to ignore the suspicion that monetary incentives may be a factor in care decisions, and it's hard not to want a system that could reward doctors equally well for performing an equally effective nonsurgical approach.

One interesting study showed how quickly even small incentives can change physician practice. A study of doctors at a large chain of walk-in clinics (eighty walk-in centers in six states) showed that doctors "performed about 20% more tests and x-rays after the owners began letting them keep part of the fees their patients paid."[34]

Coincidental?

Possibly—but again, that's not the way to bet.

PHYSICIAN PAY ISN'T THE PROBLEM—IT'S PHYSICIAN-CREATED EXPENSE!

How big a problem is the direct cost of physician care? Nowhere nearly as big as the overall impact of physician decisions.

Physicians make at least 80 to 90 percent of all health care decisions, so their practice styles drive the system. Their direct personal compensation, after overhead and expenses, probably runs only about 12 to 15 percent of the total health care bill in America. That's clearly not the lion's share of costs. Their incomes are increasing more rapidly than inflation by a significant margin, but even that increase isn't a truly significant problem.

The overwhelming problem is that the decisions they make create massive other costs within the system. Physician decisions made in favor of more extensive care significantly increase the overall cost of care for each patient.

Before discussing that impact in more detail, let's look at how much money physicians make in this country.

It is true that U.S. physicians make significantly more money than physicians in other Western countries. By way of comparison, a family practitioner in the United States makes about $120,000 per year.[35] That same doctor would make $76,800 in Canada[36] and $58,275 in Great Britain.[37] The difference for specialty areas is even more pronounced. A cardiovascular surgeon in the United States might make $292,000 per year, according to the American Group Practice Association.[38] That same doctor in Canada would average $146,000,[39] and the British surgeon would make roughly $67,599.[40]

These income levels—high as they are—would actually be a very reasonable price to pay for top-quality medical care if the overall result of that care was an efficient health care delivery system providing the most appropriate level of care. It's easy to pay physicians well if the net result is great care and overall efficiency.

Unfortunately, that's not the way it works in American health care today. Physicians are well paid, but the cost impact of their

care decisions is becoming unaffordable—and fee-for-service payment incentives are largely to blame. As an example of the lever-
aged impact that physicians have on total health costs, consider
the common medical procedure myringotomy, or as mothers refer
to it, "ear tubes." When a child has repeated ear infections, a
physician is often faced with a choice between continued use of
antibiotics (with an office visit fee of roughly $35 to $70 going to the
doctor) or performing a myringotomy in the hospital at a charge
of $500.

Clearly the ear-tube surgery pays the doctor more. There is a
significant body of evidence among physicians that not all ear-tube
operations currently being done need to be done and that continued antibiotic use would be safer and less expensive.

For the sake of argument, let's assume that a physician is motivated by the fee difference and performs the surgery unnecessarily.
What is the total cost impact of that decision?

For starters, there is the difference between the $35 to $70 con-
sultative fee and the $500 surgery fee. Then, there are postsurgery
visits, which a doctor may or may not include in the surgery fee,
depending on the degree that he or she unbundles fees. *The big
difference is the cost of the hospitalization!* Many doctors hospitalize their
patients for this procedure. A two-day hospital stay could easily
cost the insurer (and, ultimately, the consumer) another $2,000 to
$3,000 in a moderately priced hospital.

Also, the child's parents will probably take at least one day off
from work to be with their child on the day of surgery and may
need to take another half day off to bring the child home, so their
employers will lose a day or two of wages for at least one parent.

In any case, the *minimal* additional cost impact of the doctor's
decision to hospitalize and operate rather than treat the child
medically will be roughly $2,300, not counting the parents' wages
their employer lost. (That number, of course, would be offset to
some small degree by the savings that result from not prescribing
drugs otherwise needed to treat the child and by any time lost
when parents bring a child to the clinic for subsequent ear infections.)

The point is that while doctors personally take home only a very small piece of the total health care dollar, the decisions they make as a result of the fee-for-service incentives they have to increase their personal revenue have a cascading and multiplying effect on other providers and expenses.

The real cost of the doctor's decision to do unnecessary surgery isn't the additional money we pay directly to that doctor—it's the cost of the tests, equipment, surgery unit, and subsequent hospitalization. Those fees dwarf the doctor's personal revenue increase, even though that revenue increase is significant to the doctor. In cases where the procedure isn't clearly needed or useful, we would actually be miles ahead to pay doctors the full surgical fee for *not* doing the surgery in order to save the hospital expenses. (In this particular example, the doctor personally probably gets to keep only half of the surgery fee, $250. The rest of the surgery bill goes to his or her clinic's overhead expenses. The total bill for the procedure, however, includes the full $500 fee plus a $2,000 to $3,000 hospital bill and all of the miscellaneous related expenses.)

Ear tubes are a small example. The list of optional surgeries and optional treatments is almost endless, and the same factors are at play in most of them.

No reform of the system will succeed that doesn't take the leveraging impact of physician decisions into consideration.

MALPRACTICE REFORM

Some physicians point to malpractice premiums and the need to practice "defensive medicine" as a major cause of health care cost increases and as a major factor in care decisions. It is true that malpractice is a problem. The cost of malpractice coverage in this country is significant and on the rise. In 1988, roughly $6 billion was spent on malpractice premiums, a number that equaled only about 1 percent of the total health care cost in this country for that year.[41] (It is estimated, by the way, that only 40 percent of this money ever gets to injured patients; the rest goes to lawyers, insurers, and the courts.)

The cost of malpractice insurance is very unevenly distributed and weighs most heavily on physicians who do procedures such as delivering babies or performing surgery that lend themselves to malpractice awards by juries. For some medical specialties, malpractice premiums now exceed all other expenses of doing business. In other practices, malpractice premiums are relatively low. Although malpractice premiums (and suits) comprise only 1 percent of the total health care picture, they represent up to 50 percent of the costs of practice for some medical specialties and procedures. That impact has changed the practice of medicine in some very counterproductive ways. For example, in some geographic areas, malpractice premium costs have driven a large number of family practitioners out of the business of delivering babies because the additional malpractice premiums they have to pay if they deliver babies are so high.[42] This particular development has multiple impacts because, as I mentioned earlier, it not only makes family practice a less desirable specialty area for medical students, it also increases the cost of births since obstetricians have largely replaced family practitioners as "baby deliverers" and OBs tend to charge more for the service.

DEFENSIVE MEDICINE IS BOTH COSTLY AND PROFITABLE

An even greater financial impact than the 1 percent of total costs created by malpractice premiums undoubtedly results from the defensive medicine that is created by the fear of malpractice suits. Doctors often perform unnecessary tests and even unnecessary procedures in order to avoid the risk of losing a malpractice suit if a more medically appropriate approach simply proves to be "unlucky." Unnecessary procedures that are done for the sole purpose of avoiding malpractice suits are estimated by the AMA to cost us an additional $12 to $14 billion each year.[43] Some estimate this cost to be much higher.

Reform in the area of malpractice liability is clearly appropriate. But to be realistic, it's also very difficult to estimate how much of what is now labeled defensive medicine would disappear with malpractice reform. Defensive medicine in a fee-for-service environment—again, not entirely coincidentally—tends to be profitable medicine for providers. Physicians and other care providers have grown to depend on many of the revenues that result from what they call defensive medicine. If malpractice reform were to occur, it's very likely that the providers would still retain as much of the defensive style of medicine as possible to maintain the revenue. It's probably safe to say that malpractice reform might not have anywhere near the impact that its advocates project until providers are given a payment approach that rewards efficiency rather than volume.

PREPAYMENT INCENTIVES FOR PHYSICIANS

"What kind of payment approaches reward efficiency?" you might ask. The best way to reward efficiency and not volume is to prepay teams of physicians a fixed amount of money per patient to meet all of the medical needs of the patient. That general approach is referred to as "prepayment," and the payments are generally called "capitation" because they are paid "per capita" or per person, rather than "per service." Prepayment now has decades of experience behind it—and it works.

My first exposure to the direct impact of financial incentives on care delivery came when I was involved in starting an HMO in the mid-1970s. In one area of town, we had one thousand patients whose care was being reimbursed at a particular clinic on a fee-for-service basis. The use of inpatient hospital days for these patients slightly exceeded nine hundred days in the previous year, a number that was clearly excessive. When we switched the reimbursement plan for that clinic from a fee-for-service approach to a capitation plan, in which we paid the doctors a flat per capita amount of money to provide both hospital and medical care to the same one thousand people, the doctors *immediately* became more efficient and appropriate users of hospital care. The transformation took about sixty days. The hospital utilization for those one thousand people dropped from nine hundred days to five hundred days in one year, and that lower number persisted and even decreased significantly over time. Was the timing of the payment change and the hospital-use decrease coincidental? I think not.

Like all of their medical peers in the same community, the doctors at that clinic had traditionally simply ignored the issue of hospital costs since their income was based on their own fee schedule, not on the efficiency of the care they provided. They weren't alone in that regard. At that time, the average hospital-utilization rate per one thousand people across the country was also about nine hundred days.

Most fee-for-service doctors, we found in a study we did at that time, had little or no sense of the costs of the hospital care their patients were using. Again, that makes sense because those costs were not related to their own costs of doing business. Therefore, they had no financial incentive to use hospital care conservatively and efficiently.

In fact, the doctors, ironically, had a strong market-driven business incentive actually to waste hospital dollars since their patients wanted longer stays in many cases—whether or not those longer stays were medically needed. The patients were insulated from the cost of that unnecessary care by their insurance coverage, so wasteful care prevailed as the doctors conformed their practices to the wishes of their customers.

Again, it makes sense.

But at our HMO, the newly accountable doctors, who were now responsible for the first time ever for the hospital costs of their patients, thought about those costs and acted accordingly. They became more conservative users of hospital services: performing tests in their offices, discharging patients earlier, and making better decisions about the necessity and timing of admissions. They stopped doing Friday admissions for Monday surgery, for example, except in cases where the patient had an actual medical need for those days in the hospital. The doctors suddenly became aware of the cost impact of wasteful care when the dollar impact of that waste landed squarely on them, rather than on the insurer.

Once the doctors became aware of the total cost impact of their decisions, and once they were in a position where they could keep any excess capitation payments as a reward for efficiency but had to pay for any excess care out of their own clinic's bank account, they quickly became more efficient.

Over the years, I've seen that same experience repeated time after time, with providers becoming much more efficient as soon as they were given a direct financial incentive to be efficient. It can be done. I know from personal experience that it works and works quickly. In fact, it can work even more effectively today than it did back in those historic days of HMO development because we now have more sophisticated tools to use to make care both higher quality and much more efficient. In those days, all we could do was eliminate obvious waste in the use of hospital days and unnecessary tests.

The science of capitation has also progressed significantly since those early days. Modern capitation approaches put the doctors at less financial risk and focus that risk on issues over which the doctor has more direct control.

HOSPITALIZATION IS NOT WITHOUT RISK

For those of you who are wondering if the patients received lower-quality care as the result of their lower hospital usage, be assured that what was eliminated was waste—days of hospital care for which there was no medical reason. Those were, for the most part, "convenience" days for the doctors and patients, and that's a level of convenience we cannot afford.

It also bears mention that unnecessary hospital days represent more than a financial problem; they also represent a lower quality of care and a health risk to patients. A four-year, $3.1 million study done by researchers from Harvard University showed that 3.7 percent of all admissions studied were injured by the hospitals after admission and that 14 percent of those patients who were injured by the hospitals died.[44]

WASTEFUL NONSYSTEM APPROACH TO CARE

Perhaps the biggest single negative impact of the fee-for-service medical payment system is that it encourages the continuation of the current wasteful and redundant medical care delivery environment. American health care today is delivered by literally millions of independent health care profit centers, each "suboptimizing" its role in health care delivery. Fee-for-service reimbursement does not pay teams of providers for creating quality and efficiency, and therefore providers do not work as teams with those goals in mind. Because payment to care providers is made by the government and by insurers for "units of care," the health care business entities that exist, such as solo practitioners, clinics, hospitals, and pharmacists, only need to be able to provide units of care (and bill for them) to survive and thrive.

The result is a nonsystem, with no accountability for care outcomes, no tracking of performance, and no financial incentive to work together to create and standardize best practices and care protocols.

That means that we are delivering the medical science of the 1990s in the medical organizational structure of the 1940s—a bad fit, at best.

We continue to deliver care in this country through literally millions of care sites. These care sites vary widely in the quality and efficiency of their care. Rather than receive care through teams of providers working together to create the very best care approaches—each focused on the outcomes of the care being delivered—we have an inconsistent, independent approach with no guarantees that any given provider is current or skillful relative to any given health care need of a patient.

INCONSISTENT CARE

A recent study of a particular medical condition, lower urinary tract infection, illustrates the result of this nonsystem of care.[45] One hundred thirty-five private-practice doctors were asked how they would treat this particular condition. Nearly eighty-two different treatment approaches resulted—some very good and some not good at all. The cost of the approaches varied from negligible to $250 per case, with the more appropriate and effective care often costing significantly less than the most expensive care.

The current payment system does nothing to improve that amazing inconsistency in practice. In fact, every one of these eighty-two approaches was reimbursable under standard insurance contracts.

What does this tell us? It says that our care system is inefficient, inconsistent, and not focused in any organized way on achieving the best possible results. U.S. private-practice doctors treat their patients based on often outdated training or on the most recent article they can remember on a given topic. If they read the article a while ago or if the training has become obsolete in the years since they received it, then the care may not be up-to-date or appropriate.

This inadvertent medical obsolescence occurs because medicine is changing at a rapid pace and there isn't any formal, functional structure for most physicians that keeps them up-to-date. Unless they are part of a university group or a multispecialty group practice with good internal quality and educational programs, the continuing education process is, at best, hit-or-miss and, at worst, nonexistent.

Since the science of medicine changes almost daily, it is critical that doctors become part of a system or process that keeps them current on new developments and that measures the key outcomes of their care so that care can be continuously improved.

It's also going to be increasingly important to have doctors and hospitals functioning as vertically integrated teams, rather than as independent and sometimes inappropriately competing entities.

I visited a West Coast hospital a while ago and walked across a skyway to an attached—but independent—clinic. I saw an MRI machine at each end of that skyway. That's two separate million-dollar pieces of equipment. Both machines were underutilized, but each was profitable for its owner.

That, clearly, was a waste of the total health care dollar. That community should not be paying for two MRIs, but it is because the marketplace allows (and even encourages) that type of profit-driven duplication to happen. In the best of all possible worlds, those two organizations would be linked in a way that caused them to make more money and deliver better and less expensive care with a single, appropriately utilized MRI.

In the very best of all possible worlds, the decision to purchase an MRI ought to be based on the improved health care outcomes it will generate for patients, not on the improved revenue stream it can create for providers of care. The amount of technology purchased should be based on the health needs of the community, rather than the profitability of a clinic.

DOCTOR BASHING ISN'T THE ANSWER—OR THE POINT

The point of this chapter is not to say that physicians as a group act unethically (driven by greed and their economic self-interest) or to suggest that American medicine is not the best in the world. For those who can afford it, it usually is.

It's also plain to see that the traditional "Marcus Welby" type of commitment to the patient is alive and well.

The dedication of the men and women who go into pediatrics, family practice, and general internal medicine in the face of over-whelming financial incentives to select other specialty areas, for example, speaks well for the commitment of these physicians to the patient. A great many of the specialists who do the high-tech procedures referred to earlier also deserve to be called heroes: working long hours in often physically taxing circumstances to serve their patients. I, personally, would not ever be able to handle either the physical or mental rigor of long, complicated surgery,

much less the tension and pressure. I've watched surgical procedures being performed, and I marvel at the surgeon's dexterity,
stamina, and skill. Doctors work hard and often accomplish miracles.

The real point of this chapter is to explain how the economics
and the current structure of the current system work against medical efficiency. We do not reward our caregivers for cures, for
improving health outcomes, or for delivering efficient care. Instead, we rather crudely reward them for performing volumes of
services. When our goal is to buy cures, we shouldn't be paying for
something else. We need to reward teams of providers for the
quality and outcomes of the care. We should not focus on encouraging independent providers or unrelated units of service.

As you will see in the following chapters, the problem of perverse and counterproductive incentives is not confined to the
medical profession. The many pieces of our complex health care
delivery system do not work together. Rather, each health care
business unit works in its own economic self-interest to maximize
its own piece of the health care dollar. Results of that perversely
motivated nonstructure include inefficiency, waste, and poorer
quality care than we should be getting, given the amount of money
we spend in this country on health care.

It's particularly frustrating to observe this situation in the context of the thirty to forty million uninsured Americans who, in the
midst of this wealth of health care, do not have access to basic
health coverage. It's clear that the current system, with its perverse
financial incentives, does not address this troubling problem ade-
quately.

The observations about the impact of fee-for-service incentives
on care are not a new discovery. The relationship between the way
we pay our doctors and the resultant behavior has been observed
for some time. In the introduction to *The Doctor's Dilemma,* George
Bernard Shaw noted,

> It is not the fault of our doctors that the medical service of the
> community, as at present provided for, is a murderous absurd-

ity. That any sane nation, having observed that you could provide for the supply of bread by giving bakers a pecuniary interest in baking for you, should go on to give a surgeon a pecuniary interest in cutting off your leg, is enough to make one despair of political humanity. But that is precisely what we have done. And the more appalling the mutilation, the more the mutilator is paid. He who corrects the ingrowing toe-nail receives a few shillings: he who cuts your inside out receives hundreds of guineas, except when he does it on a poor person for practice.[46]

The challenge we need to face is how better to align our payments with our goals so that doctors can focus on efficiency, on quality, and on cures and can be freed from the indignity of trolling for warts.

Chapter 3

HOSPITALS

Hospitals in America are significantly less efficient than they could and should be, and the primary cause of their inefficiency is, as with doctors, the way we have chosen to reimburse and capitalize them.

That fact of economic life has become increasingly evident to observers of the hospital situation. The American Hospital Association, a strong advocate for hospitals' interests, acknowledged in a recent report entitled "Renewing the U.S. Health Care System" that major problems exist and that "to be blunt, the key word is waste—not 'inefficiency' or 'misallocation' of resources, but *waste*!"[1]

Why is this? And how did it come to be?

Hospitals are wasteful in large part because they are rewarded financially for attracting doctors to their staffs, rather than for delivering efficient or effective care to patients.

Like physicians, hospitals are usually paid by the government and private payers on a fee-for-service basis. Like physicians, they are paid for units of care and, again like physicians, they are often very good at both increasing and itemizing those units of care in ways that maximize their revenue.

Also like physicians, hospitals tend not to be rewarded in any tangible way for achieving, recording, or reporting positive outcomes from the care they deliver.

Unlike physicians, however, hospitals usually do not have direct access to the patient marketplace. For the most part (and there are exceptions, such as emergency rooms or special care programs), hospitals get their patients from doctors. In the United States, patients typically do not choose hospitals, patients choose doctors. Doctors then choose hospitals.

That simple fact of market reality means that hospitals must attract doctors in order to succeed. How do hospitals do that? With a great deal of energy and creativity. They work hard to recruit doctors to their own staff and to the staff of medical groups that use their hospital. They help finance new doctors who are starting practices and will use their hospital. They create great physician lounges, dining rooms, and related amenities to give the doctors a sense of comfort and convenience. And, in a way that drives health care costs up at an accelerating rate, hospitals compete for doctors by using hospital money to create medical workshops such as surgeries and laboratories that doctors can use to enhance their personal revenues.

The battles between hospitals to persuade physicians or medical groups to switch their loyalties from one institution to another can be as bloody as anything that occurs in U.S. business today, as hospitals offer their target physicians and medical groups clinic space, the newest technology, various support services, intensive flattery, and even joint-venture status for potentially lucrative care programs. In cities where there are multiple hospitals, if you checked into a typical hospital war room, where the administrators meet privately to plot out their operational strategy, you would probably see lists of their target physicians as well as defensive lists that identify which of their own physicians may be in the process of being lured away by some other hospital.

This process, unfortunately, consumes much of the creativity and energy of hospital management teams and adds very little to either the cost efficiency or quality of health care.

I've heard hospital administrators celebrate the successful wooing of a particularly attractive medical practice into their hospital with the gusto most of us reserve for a hole in one or a long-awaited addition to the family.

In that competitive process, a lot of health care dollars get spilled. We end up with a number of full-service, technology-laden, highly competitive hospitals in a given geographic area that would be better and more efficiently served with a few hospital centers of excellence in key specialty areas. Every hospital in a multihospital town does not need an autologous bone-marrow transplant program, for example, if one or two programs could cover the needs of the entire community at a lower cost. But if every hospital wants to attract and maintain its own set of oncologists, they may find that it's a better overall financial decision for each of them to build a redundant transplant unit. The alternative in today's care environment may well be for the hospital to lose its key oncologists to a competing hospital that has such a unit.

Since fee-for-service payment approaches typically do not attempt to influence either overall health system efficiency or quality, the hospitals can build their redundant units and simply bill their various payers at a per-procedure cost that meets (and probably exceeds) the revenue need created by the expense of building and operating those units.

The charges for these types of programs can vary widely between institutions of comparable structure but different market conditions. I've seen hospitals in a town with several bone-marrow units charge as much as $200,000 per case, while other hospitals in towns where there is only one bone-marrow program can charge less than $100,000 for the same (or better) care. The difference is that the single-hospital site can operate at full capacity.

A GOLDEN AGE FOR HOSPITALS

To understand how the current hospital environment came into existence, it might be useful to get a brief historical perspective. Until the 1970s, hospitals operated in a world of plenty. They had access to large amounts of capital from the Hill-Burton Act of 1946, and they could build or expand their facilities fairly freely with government grants and very low interest money. The rules for proving "need" for that money were pretty lax. (I know of a hospital, in fact, that used cheap capital to build an entire wing years ago that effectively doubled the hospital's size and then immediately mothballed the entire wing because it wasn't needed. I'm not sure if it has been used to this day.)

At the same time, insurers and the government were either accepting each hospital's charges at face value without question or, better yet, paying the hospitals on a cost-plus basis.

Think about the situation: Hospitals could build or expand almost at will with cheap or free money, the major payers paid them on a cost-plus or full-fee basis, and no one questioned their fee schedules or the use of services by their doctors or patients.

Financially, it was a golden age for hospitals, and they are still recovering. The major role of the hospital CEO in that happy era was to recruit medical staff and keep both the doctors and the hospital board politically happy. The financial situation pretty much handled itself. Generally, hospitals were not all that competitive with each other since there were more than enough patient days to go around and costs were irrelevant to the marketplace. The interhospital world was convivial and pleasant.

The End of the Golden Age

Then, in the 1970s and 1980s, that golden age started to fall apart. Cost-plus reimbursement disappeared. Medicare, Medicaid, and various forms of competing health plans began to insist on hospital discounts. Some of the government discounts were so deep that they created, in effect, a hidden tax on other payers, whose prices went up to offset the government's underpayments. Even the Blues began to put caps on the hospitals' rate increases. Certificate-of-need requirements for hospital development and expansion came and went. Free expansion money disappeared (replaced, however, to some degree with low-interest, tax-free bonding opportunities).

In some areas, for-profit hospital chains emerged to put pressure on local, not-for-profit hospitals for the most lucrative categories of patients. Hospitals found themselves competing for HMO and PPO patients through discounts in a number of major markets.

The emergence of fee-for-service-based, free-standing surgery centers in many markets also put pressure on the hospitals by drawing away some of their most profitable patients. Rural hospitals increasingly found themselves overbuilt, with a decreasing patient and population base, shrinking lengths of stay, and increasing percentages of patients who were either uninsured or covered by deeply discounted government programs such as Medicare and Medicaid.

The hospital world changed in two decades from a world in which hospitals had to be downright stupid to lose money to a world in which many hospital CEOs had to be first-rate entrepreneurs to make money and survive.

America, however, has never had a shortage of entrepreneurs. The hospital industry, faced with the financial pressures and realities of the 1980s, clearly found its share.

HOSPITAL MARKETING EFFORTS—FRILLS AND TECHNOLOGY

Hospitals began to market themselves aggressively to both patients and doctors. I can still remember the first hospital "birthing unit" I saw that offered a hotel-quality suite, complete with soft music, a double bed (so the father could stay in the hospital with the new mother and baby), and postbirth champagne for the new parents. The hospital's motivation for creating those units obviously wasn't improved quality of care, but, rather, greater enjoyment of the process for the patients and, as a result, improved patient volume for the hospital.

Since the birthing unit patients were insulated from the costs of the hospital stay by their insurance coverage, they didn't take issue with the hospital about the nonmedical costs of these programs. Neither, for the most part, did the insurers, particularly since the actual costs of building those units were often not itemized in hospital bills but were hidden somewhere in the overall hospital charges.

On a grander scale, many hospitals also turned to technology to generate additional revenue. Hospital marketing staffs creatively realized that they could recruit specialists to their medical staffs and find ways around the price-constraining basic-care contracts they were increasingly forced to sign with the Blues, HMOs, PPOs, and even some insurers by creating new, technology-dependent care programs. Since most managed care contracts typically applied only to routine care, many hospitals invested heavily in programs offering "nonroutine" care in order to generate revenue that was not limited by any contractual pricing agreements.

Technology expansion has been explosive. Hospitals have made massive investments in CT scanners, MRI equipment, surgical lasers, and other expensive and high-tech programs that generate high medical fees and patient flow.

One of the reasons that we offer the highest quality of care in the world for most of our citizens (when they have severe illnesses) is that equipment. (This book isn't intended to be critical, at all, of true technological enhancements and progress. My own aged grandmother has had a much improved quality of life over the past several years because of repeated laser surgery for her eyes, for example.) The problem, however, is that our current fee-for-service reimbursement system allows, encourages, and rewards overinvestment in that very expensive technology, and, as a result, we waste significant amounts of money on underutilized, redundant, and extremely expensive equipment and programs.

As McManis Associates, a highly regarded hospital and health care consulting organization, noted in a supplement to *Health Care Competition Week*, "Not only do we continue to have an overabundance of inpatient acute care capacity, we also now have more individual hospitals duplicating capacity in other areas in their quest for survival. The result is still higher costs and greater underutilization of capacity. Hospitals become caught in spiraling cost increases as they spend more to expand services and buy technology. The high costs of expansion are eventually passed on to consumers."[2]

THE HOSPITAL ARMS RACE

Hospitals aren't overjoyed with their situation. In order to survive, entrepreneurial hospital executives make the investments, create the programs, and, I suspect, often wonder how they managed to stray from their original career goal of providing high-quality health care in a world where they compete with each other for doctors and revenue by creating expensive and redundant programs in a country where millions of people can't afford even basic care.

Gordon Sprenger, president of HealthSpan Hospitals in Minneapolis and a past chair of the Voluntary Hospitals of America (VHA), expressed a common wish when he said, "Perhaps it is too difficult right now to go back and try to change what is already in place, but maybe we can start changing future behavior. Let's stop the 'medical arms race.' "[3]

Other hospital CEOs agree. A Louis Harris and Associates survey taken of 251 CEOs of larger hospitals asked what they would exchange for high occupancy and more predictable reimbursement. Nearly two thirds (62 percent) were willing to accept more stringent limits on capital spending for new capacity. Just over half (51 percent) were willing to accept stricter limits on costly new technology, and 53 percent were willing to accept a significant reduction in the number of beds in the hospital.[4] Interestingly and sadly, 82 percent of the hospital CEOs also believed that rationing of expensive, high-tech medical services would be needed in the future, in large part to stop the "medical arms race."

Another study, by Deloitte & Touche, also indicated that hospital CEOs are generally unhappy with the role in which they find themselves. More than half of those studied said they "would leave health care if offered equivalent salaries."[5]

Hospital CEOs often find themselves under great pressure from their medical staffs. A while ago, I talked to one hospital head whose hospital already owned and operated three MRI's, each costing millions of dollars. He said that a group of private doctors practicing at his hospital had recently approached him with a business play to buy yet another MRI in a joint-venture relationship between the hospital and the doctors. The pro forma financial projections they brought to the table indicated that they believed they could drum up enough business to make the machine profitable for them and the hospital. The implied threat in their request was that they would take their offer, and their business, to another hospital if the hospital turned them down.

To put that request into perspective, we already had more then a dozen MRIs in that community of two million people. As of the date of that request, however, there were only fifteen MRIs in all of Canada.[6]

The CEO acknowledged that the equipment and the program would be completely redundant, but said that he probably would have to go along with the purchase in order to keep those members of his medical staff happy. "We are increasingly in the business of helping doctors make money," he said. "They, not the patient, are the source of our customers. We need to respond to the market that we serve."

Another hospital CEO recently told me that his hospital was spending millions to add surgery units. The request for the new units came from a private medical group who already worked at the hospital but couldn't get access to what they considered to be the prime, early-morning surgery times. The doctors weren't willing to wait until the existing surgery units opened up later in the day, so they demanded expensive new units and equipment for their own convenience.

Again, the threat was that the physicians would take their practice and move to another hospital if they couldn't get access to early surgery times. The issue wasn't quality of care or improving patient outcomes—it was keeping the physicians from shifting their practice to another hospital. The units are being built.

The net cost to the community of those types of incidents is substantial. The public will need to pay—through taxes, premiums, and direct bills—for the cost of that redundant MRI and those excess surgery units. And, for most of the day, those surgery units will sit empty, a testimonial to our current system's inefficient use of capital.

HOSPITAL COMPETITION INCREASES PRICES

As noted earlier in the case of bone-marrow transplants, one very interesting and counterintuitive result of hospital versus hospital competition for the fee-for-service dollar (and the fee-for-service doctor) is a strange and very direct relationship between the existence of competing hospitals in a given town and the cost of hospital services. In other words, when hospitals compete, prices go up. That result seems to contradict traditional economic theory, until you understand a hospital's real marketplace.

Based on traditional economic theories about monopolies, one might expect that in a one-hospital town, the single hospital would be free of competitive pricing pressure and would be able (and likely) to set its prices at high, monopoly-type levels. On the other hand, if one thinks in the context of a typical competitive marketplace, one might also suspect that the existence of a competing hospital in a given community would lead both hospitals to achieve lower costs in order to compete on price. That, in fact, does not happen in either case. Exactly the opposite result occurs. Hospital costs go up in our current fee-for-service environment when there are multiple hospitals in the same town.

The simple fact is that hospitals compete for doctors, not for patients, and cost is irrelevant to doctors. The factors that are most attractive and relevant to doctors drive hospital costs up—not down—because the doctors are both insulated from any negative market-related impact of their cost decisions and strongly rewarded by the current payment system for actions that result in increased costs.

Once that dynamic is understood, the relationship between hospital competition and hospital cost situation makes perfect sense.

In a one-hospital town, the hospital CEO is freed from the competitive pressures to outdo the next hospital by creating expensive programs and purchasing expensive technology. In towns with two or more hospitals, however, a given hospital's doctors consistently have the negotiating leverage of being able to move from one hospital to another, so they can force hospitals to create expensive programs whether or not they are needed by the community.

The interesting and perverse result of hospital competition, according to one study, is that "hospital costs are 20 to 21 percent higher where competition is heaviest and six percent higher in two hospital towns over hospitals with no neighbors."[7] A similar study concluded that hospitals in multihospital towns competed relative to "who has . . . the fanciest equipment."

Again, the patient is insulated from the costs of this medical arms race by insurance. And insurance doesn't get involved in issues of care-system efficiency or unnecessary capital investments. Hospitals are also insulated from the total cost impact of those decisions because they are not now part of any team of caregivers who are—as a team—accountable for the total cost of care. As independent profit centers, they only have to be able to charge a fee for each service that exceeds their own cost of creating that service. Fee-for-service insurance allows this to happen. The inefficiencies created by the doctor-focused competitive strategies of the hospitals are therefore financed by the insurers, employers, and government programs that pay the bill for the redundant services. For the most part, the hospital's doctor-focused competitive strategies create very little added value for either the hospital's product or the overall community.

The ability of hospitals to evade the constraints of managed care contracts and to achieve fee-based revenue growth by creating new imaging, treatment, or diagnostic programs may be diminishing over time, as HMOs and PPOs increasingly dominate the marketplace. Even insurers are beginning to contract for some care, and the largest insurers are making commitments to managed care in a number of markets. As the various forms of managed care grow, the portion of the market that pays billed charges in full to the hospitals and doesn't question the appropriateness of care will correspondingly shrink. By the mid-1990s, this trend will force already beleaguered hospitals in many markets to seek new approaches to maintain their status and profit margins.

The hospitals' strategic dilemma is compounded by another powerful trend—the increasing ability of physicians to deliver high-tech care in nonhospital settings. That trend—coupled with shorter hospital stays for certain types of increasingly less invasive surgeries—will result in hospitals facing major reductions in the number of patient days for which they can charge fees. By the mid-1990s, many hospitals will be functioning as intensive care units—while well-equipped clinics perform many surgeries and procedures on an outpatient basis. In that context, the need for our current hospital bed infrastructure will shrink dramatically.

That presents an interesting challenge for hospitals as they develop their long-range plans. Currently, hospitals have revenue, patient volume, and capital. They will soon have less of each of those if current trends continue. By the mid-nineties, they will have tougher payers and fewer patients and they may be facing major capital shortages and controls.

HOSPITALS AS COMMODITIES, COMPONENTS, OR CORES OF CARE SYSTEMS

As these pressures increase, hospitals will need to choose between being "commodities," "components," or "cores" for the HMO-like care systems that probably will emerge in the 1990s. As commodities they would continue to sell services to the care systems without becoming a part of the care system itself. More conservative hospitals may attempt that strategy in order to maintain their current status as independent entities and profit centers.

Other hospitals will probably choose to become components— or integral parts of managed care systems—and, if the market responds favorably, they will have strong incentives to become efficient as part of those systems. Those hospitals will stop being separate and independent businesses or "profit centers" in the larger health care economy and will instead become "cost centers" as departments or care units within larger, vertically integrated care systems.

Other hospitals will choose a more independent, hospital-centered approach and will take advantage of their current credibility and capital to form their own managed care systems. Those hospitals will purchase clinics, hire doctors, and attempt to sell their services directly to both governmental and private payers. They will, in effect, become the core element of a new generation of HMOs as we currently know them.

Other hospitals will simply fight the trend and may attempt to turn back the clock by seeking legislative or congressional relief from the disciplines of cost containment, negotiated contracts, or market forces. Those more reactionary hospitals will probably favor a single-payer approach to national health insurance, in which the government is the only insurer and either pays providers on a fee-for-service basis or awards each provider a budget as a way to freeze the current health care delivery system solidly into place. That approach would enable the hospitals to avoid the rigors of care management and system redesign and allow them to make their current inefficiencies permanent. Like the physicians who see a fee-for-service-based single-payer system as the best way of guaranteeing their current income stream (allowing them to avoid real system reform), some hospitals have already started supporting reform approaches that will, in actuality, simply maintain the status quo. Most hospitals, however, are more progressive than that and look forward to a day when they are rewarded more for serving patients than for increasing physician revenues.

The more innovative hospitals will also look for ways to band together to create market strength. The better-structured hospital systems of the 1990s will be much more selective in their use of capital and creation of programs, and—instead of running duplicate programs in every hospital—they will designate individual hospitals within each system as "centers of excellence" for specific diseases and conditions.

This is a step forward relative to eliminating capital redundancy, but it will not prevent other systems in the same geographic area from creating duplicate centers of excellence for their own networks.

Even with no market reform or health care restructuring of any kind, the hospitals of the mid-1990s will face major pressures from new technology and care patterns. As the newest technology reduces the length of hospital stays for common procedures, as increasing numbers of procedures can be done on an outpatient basis, as births become a one- or (at most) two-day stay, as lower-cost skilled nursing facilities become the treatment site of choice for patients with chronic conditions whose care doesn't require a full set of hospital services, and as hospices increasingly become the preferred care facility for the terminally ill, hospitals will see a major shrinkage in use by the mid-1990s.

This means that the hospital of the future will be high-tech and short-stay and will be serving only the most acute cases. It also means that we have far too many hospital beds in use today.

How serious is the problem of hospital competition, fueled by our current fee-for-service reimbursement approach?

A study by American Health Care Systems in May of 1990 calculated that there are approximately 194,000 excess hospital beds in this country. There are an additional 136,000 beds that are usually unoccupied but are used during peak periods, according to previous government reports.[8]

The study indicates that the number of beds continues to drop; about twelve thousand beds closed each year in 1988 and 1989. That still left the occupancy levels of U.S. community hospitals at only 64.9 percent for 1989. In my own marketplace, where hospitals have had to face the full brunt of managed care for the past two decades, we've seen nearly a dozen hospital closings in the past ten years. HMOs and PPOs have reduced hospital admissions, shortened the length of stay for most conditions, and generally made more efficient use of hospitals.

As a result, according to Don Wegmiller, retired president of the Twin City–based Health One hospital system, there is "much less need for inpatient hospital care today than there was in 1980 or 1970." Approximately one million fewer inpatient hospital days were needed in 1991, compared to 1981, in spite of a growing and aging population. According to Wegmiller, "That's about ten 400-bed hospitals taken out of the system."[9]

At least partially as a result, Twin City health care costs are the lowest of any major city in the country, according to several recent surveys. According to one national survey taken by H. Foster Higgins & Company,[10] the premiums paid by employers in Minnesota averaged nearly $600 a year less per employee than the national average. Another survey, done by Milliman and Robertson, supported the H. Foster Higgins & Company study. The Milliman and Robertson study looked at the fifteen largest cities in the United States and also concluded that the health premium costs in the Twin Cities were the lowest of any market studied.[11]

These numbers represent real savings for the marketplace, but they are clearly not sufficient to claim victory over health care costs.

In our market, because we still have a significant level of nonmanaged care, we still have hospitals investing heavily in new programs designed to take a market share from other hospitals. We have arm's length negotiations between health plans and hospitals, with each party attempting to improve its position relative to the other. We have inefficiencies that result from the lack of joint goal setting and program planning between clinics and hospitals. And we have redundant care programs that run at half capacity and full cost.

These problems are occurring in a setting where managed care is the dominant market force because we have not finished the process of vertical integration and because a significant portion of the marketplace continues to use fee-for-service reimbursement. In other settings, however, where pure fee-for-service reimbursement is dominant, even greater problems exist.

If you doubt my assessment of the role that financial decisions play in hospital planning, go to your nearest bookstore or library and scan through some hospital magazines. You won't find many articles about care. The articles are about the business of being a hospital.

I subscribe to several of those magazines in order to keep in touch with hospital thinking on financial issues. One of my favorite examples of hospital strategic thinking comes from one of them. The purpose of this particular magazine is to help hospital executives improve their institution's market position. Under the headline CARDIAC ER CAN INCREASE ADMISSIONS, PROFITS, IMAGE, a recent article explained how hospitals can achieve a profitable increase in cardiology admissions by creating a special emergency program targeted at "chest pain."

After spending several pages outlining both the low investment required to create such a program and the potentially large profits that can be generated, the article issues a warning to the hospital executive: "The market advantage of a chest pain ER is likely to diminish over time because other providers in each market will create comparable programs." However, the article then reassures the reader that this ultimate loss of market share shouldn't discourage hospitals from developing such programs because the interim profits will be sufficient to justify the investment. The article concludes by saying, "A chest pain ER is worth doing if only to save the lives of patients suffering from heart attacks . . . but it is also a tremendous way to generate incremental profits."[12]

That reference to the lives of patients was *the first and only* mention in the entire article of any benefit to the patients. Saving patient lives is listed as a *by-product* of the program.

Enough said.

Hospitals shouldn't have to focus their energy on recruiting medical staff and increasing the volumes of services. They should be able to focus their energy on improving the quality of care, improving health care outcomes, and improving efficiency. When we create an incentive system that actually rewards outcomes and efficiency, we will make hospital administrators much happier as a profession and we will get the outcomes we want.

Right now, we get what we pay for.

Chapter 4

TECHNOLOGY AND
DRUGS—MIRACLES AND PROFITS

It's interesting to review some recent numbers comparing Canada's use of high-tech care and sophisticated medical procedures with the use of those same approaches in this country. A study published in the March 1993 *New England Journal of Medicine* showed that 68 percent of U.S. heart patients received "imaging services" versus only 35 percent of Canadian patients. Thirty-one percent of the U.S. patients had surgery, compared to only 12 percent in Canada.[1]

The study also showed that 23 percent of the U.S. patients died, compared to 22 percent of the Canadian patients.

One has to ask if we receive proper value for all the additional money that is spent in the United States on the X-rays and the surgery or if many of the care decisions made here are, perhaps, related more to provider revenue and the availability of excess technology, rather than the patient's well-being.

Until further studies are done, we really don't know the answer to that question. The science of medicine changes daily. New drugs, new technologies, new uses for current technologies, new techniques, and new procedures are reported almost continuously in the professional journals and even in the mass media.

To a great extent, these changes represent progress, with progress defined as better health care outcomes for the patients who receive the services.

The problem is that these changes also represent increased health care costs. The new technologies, drugs, and procedures sometimes add very little value to care, but they almost invariably cost the public more than the treatments they replace or supplement.

In fact, changes in the practice of medicine are the primary factor in the rapid inflation in health care costs today. These changes take place at all levels of care—from primary care through the most sophisticated, high-tech care—and their impact is pervasive. No element of care is static.

We did a simple study in some of our medical practices a couple of years ago to ascertain the reasons for our own increasing health care costs. Our conclusion was that even in a care system that is relatively conservative in its choice of care approaches, slightly more than 50 percent of the increase in costs over a three-year period was due to changes in the practice of medicine. Those changes included new drugs, new technology, and expanded uses of existing technology for both primary and specialty care. During that period, our overall care costs increased by nearly 40 percent, a number that was significantly lower than the health care inflation rate in the country at the time, to put it in perspective. If the study was valid, and we believe it was, we could theoretically have reduced the increase in care costs by roughly 50 percent by freezing the practice of medicine during that time period.

That would have resulted in a total care cost nearly 20 percent below the actual costs that occurred.

If one ran that same ratio backward for two more years and applied it to the entire country, one could speculate that we could have reduced overall health care costs in this country by more than a third by freezing our medical practice approaches at the level of five years ago. The result of that freeze would have been a per capita health care cost that equals per capita costs in Canada today.

The result would also have been the health care approach of five years ago—a world without MRIs, Prozac, Doppler ultrasound, or arthroscopic surgery, to name a few of the technology and treatment changes that were popularized during that time span.

Freezing the health care delivery process at a given point in time clearly isn't feasible or acceptable, but the concept is interesting as a way of thinking about the cost impact that new drugs and new care approaches have on U.S. health care.

Where do these new drugs, technologies, and care approaches come from? They originate in two of the most successful, creative, energetic, and market-driven industries in the world today—the U.S. medical technology and pharmaceutical industries. While the rest of our economy has been in the doldrums, these industries have enjoyed record profits and record sales and have an extremely favorable international balance of trade that is almost unique in today's U.S. economy. By any measure of capitalistic success, these two industries are major winners.

The key questions that need to be answered are (1) Can we afford to have them win quite so handily?, (2) Do the new drugs and technologies create improved health outcomes that justify their cost?, and (3) Do some of the new drugs and technologies improve care outcomes at all?

The truth that we need to face if we want to reform health care delivery is this: At the same time that those industries have been giving us wonder drugs and miracle technologies, they have also been key players in creating a health care environment that is too often wasteful and inefficient, with excess technology and inefficient drugs used far too often in instances where less expensive alternatives would do as well or better.

Technology Creates Both Better Care and Higher Provider Revenue

The critical factor to keep in mind is that medical technology is sold both for its ability to provide improved care *and* for its ability to generate revenue for health care providers. Unfortunately, those two objectives do not always coincide.

There is no shortage of studies that help make that point. A 1991 California study of workers' compensation cases showed, for example, that when physician groups owned their own magnetic resonance imaging machine, they tended to make 68 percent more scans than a comparable sample of physicians who did *not* own an MRI.[2] At an average cost per MRI referral of more than $930, that is not an insignificant cost difference.

A recent Florida study showed similar results.[3] An analysis of Medicare data showed that in situations where physicians had a high incidence of joint-venture ownership interest in radiation therapy services, the doctors prescribed 139 radiation treatments per one thousand Medicare enrollees. That compares to only eighty-eight treatments per one thousand enrollees for a population whose physicians were not, for the most part, joint owners of such equipment.

That difference in treatment was not due to a sicker population. In fact, the cancer rate for the population of Medicare patients who received more treatments was actually about 8 percent *lower* than the cancer rate for the population that received eighty-eight treatments per one thousand people.

Another fascinating study done of insurance claims for the United Mineworkers of America showed even more dramatic results.[4] In this study, researchers found that physicians who owned imaging equipment were 1.9 times more likely to use imaging to diagnose chest pain, 3.6 times more likely to use the equipment for low back pain, and 7.7 times more likely to require an image for knee pain.

The extent to which technology purchase and use decisions are driven by financial consideration rather than patient outcome objectives is often discouraging.

I've talked to a number of hospital administrators who have been asked by private-practice physicians to enter into joint-venture purchases of high-tech equipment (such as MRIs). When

I asked the hospital administrators how often the physician's proposed plan for the equipment included any general or quantifiable target objectives for improving the quality or efficiency of care, the answer consistently was that the physician's business plans had been just that—business plans—with a focus on patient volume, revenue, and profitability, rather than care.

In other words, those plans typically do not say that "if we just had an MRI we could save sixteen more lives per year" or "we could avoid a dozen unnecessary exploratory surgeries each month." Those kinds of outcomes do happen, but they are, unfortunately, usually not the formal objective of the purchasing process.

HOSPITAL TECHNOLOGY/CAPITAL PLANS OFTEN FOCUS ON REVENUE, NOT CARE

Hospitals can't blame the focus on technology as a revenue provider on their physicians. Hospitals often take a similar approach in their own planning. I had an opportunity a short while ago to review the strategic plans and objectives of a couple of large, nationally known hospitals from widely separate states. It was interesting (and sadly confirming) to read through page after page of hospital objectives about increasing the number of patient referrals, maximizing the number of patient visits, and so forth. I found only one very brief reference in two entire plans to a single quality objective: One of the hospitals intended to create a "report to the patient" about a small list of health care outcomes that Medicare was studying in that hospital.

Other than that one lonely reference, the hospitals focused their own plans entirely on business issues.

Those hospitals are in the process of spending hundreds of millions of dollars over the next several years—much of that money earmarked to upgrade their technology—without any corporate objectives dealing with the results of their patient care.

If any hospital administrators of your acquaintance challenge that perspective and suggest that their own strategic plans focus more on care issues than business factors, please ask to see their actual strategic plan documents before assuming that I have done them a disservice.

No One Knows Exactly How Well Competing Equipment Works

Interestingly, although we spend billions of dollars in this country on health care technology, there is not a lot of data available for health care providers to use as they make their technology purchasing decisions. There aren't any good *Consumer Reports*-type comparisons that would tell a potential buyer that "mammography Machine A is as accurate and lasts twice as long, on the average, as Machine B—so it's a good deal, even at its 25 percent higher price."

Doctors don't even have good, objective information that tells them if pacemaker A has better outcomes than pacemaker B.

I had a chance to talk to a marketing person for implantable medical devices a while back and asked him if his company provided comparisons of their product with others to the surgeons who are their target market.

"No, we don't use that type of comparative data," he said, "*unless* we have a real clear example of our product's superiority. Otherwise, we expect the doctor to listen to us, then listen to the other sales pitches, and decide. It's up to the doctors to make those kinds of comparisons—not us."

I'm not sure about you, but if I someday need a pacemaker, I'd like my doctor to have a more scientific way of evaluating alternatives than the relative sales skills of each manufacturer's marketing team.

PHARMACEUTICAL SALES APPROACHES ARE LEGENDARY

The problem of uncertain benefits and unknown relative product value is magnified for pharmaceuticals. Most doctors learn about drugs from the drug companies' detail men, who haunt medical practices, giving our free samples and urging doctors to try their new products. It is one of the most amazingly comparison-devoid marketing environments in any science-related field.

The pharmaceutical companies in the United States have been raising prices regularly for the past decade. In fact, although prescription drugs amount to roughly 10 percent of the total personal-consumption expenditures in this country,[5] the rate of increase in prescription drug prices rose almost 20 percent more than medical inflation each year from 1980 to 1990. Drug manufacturers' profitability is also high. The annual return on stockholder equity is 20 percent, twice the average of other Fortune 500 companies.[6]

The drug companies have defended their cost increases by pointing to the massive research expenses associated with the development of new drugs. These costs, in fact, are high—upwards of $9 billion a year—but they are actually exceeded by the money the drug companies spend to market their products.[7]

Not only do the drug companies spend literally billions of dollars to place their names and products before the medical profession, they are also now spending $100 million a year on direct advertising to U.S. consumers to persuade consumers to ask their doctors for particular drugs.[8]

Drug companies also usually push their products without giving doctors solid, sufficient, scientific information about the relative merits of their drugs compared to others already in the market. The recent controversy about the relative merits of the clot-dissolving drugs streptokinase and tissue plasminogen activator (tPA) is one example. Streptokinase costs about $240 a dose. TPA costs $2,400 a dose. Each helps dissolve coronary clots to help save the lives of people who are having heart attacks.[9]

Studies released by the manufacturer of tPA made it appear that tPA was clearly the better, more effective choice, and thousands of physicians and hospitals switched to that higher-priced drug to save lives. Later, more objective studies compared tPA and streptokinase in a toe-to-toe comparison, and these studies indicated that streptokinase was probably the more effective treatment in most cases. More recent studies, however, seem to indicate that tPA may actually have a 1 percent better mortality rate.[10] Given the relative difference in costs between the drugs, that 1 percent advantage means that it will cost $22,000 for each additional life saved if cardiologists switch to tPA.[11] At this point, doctors are simply reading conflicting data and making their own best choices.

That's clearly not the best way to make decisions of that nature, but it's too often the way those decisions are made. In fact, the doctors who are choosing between the two drugs actually have more data than doctors usually have when choosing between other drugs for other conditions.

NEW DRUGS USUALLY ARE NOT "BETTER" DRUGS

The drug companies do not help matters much by continually bringing new drugs whose relative merit is questionable onto the market. As an example, between 1981 and 1988, U.S. drug companies brought a total of 348 new drugs to market.[12] Of that number, the FDA rated 308, or 84 percent, of these new drugs as "C-class" drugs. A C-class drug is one that works better than a placebo, but it does not necessarily work better than other drugs already on the market. At best, these drugs offer a treatment that is "therapeutically equivalent" to other drugs already available.

If the new drugs aren't better, you might ask, why are they introduced into the market? To be fair, there are some medical reasons. In some cases, patients may be allergic to a current drug and a new drug might bypass their allergic reactions. In other cases, the new drug might create fewer side effects when used in conjunction with another drug being taken by a patient who has multiple health problems.

These factors are not, however, the most common quality that these new C-class drugs share. The most common factor is that, in almost all cases, the new drug is more expensive than the old drug that it replaces. The new drug represents a marketing opportunity for the drug company, and, since new drugs typically have newer patents, they give the drug manufacturer longer-lived protection against "generic equivalents" that may be offered by other manufacturers at much lower costs when the patent on a given drug expires.

Drug company marketing efforts are legendary. As a senior executive for a company that operates pharmacies as part of our care system, I've been invited to all-expenses-paid "seminars" at world-famous golf resorts and even all-expenses-paid trips to oversea "symposiums." The working agendas for these seminars tend to be fairly brief, although the speakers are sometimes world-class. The golf and recreation time tends to be substantial.

I do not, by the way, accept any of these invitations.

We've also had a drug company offer to connect our clinics by satellite to continuously televised, high-quality health education programs in exchange for their being able to run a few infomercials about their products between programs. (We didn't do that either, but it was tempting.)

Other sales approaches used by drug companies include providing doctors with free magazines, gifts, medical retreats, and hospitality rooms at medical meetings and conventions. In some cases, the sales materials for drug companies are cleverly disguised as professional presentations. The FDA has intervened to force companies to acknowledge that supposedly objective articles written about the effects of their drugs are actually articles written by "paid agents" of the drug companies.

I could go on at length, but I hope the point is made. The current approach to marketing prescription drugs creates health care costs that are unnecessary and often wasteful. We need a better process for selecting both the technology and the drugs that we use in our health care systems. Ideally, that process will examine the therapeutic impact and cost of the drug and will create a scientifically based scorecard that providers can use to make prescribing decisions.

BETTER COMPARISON DATA IS NEEDED

This is not an academic point. When studies of comparative outcomes are done, the results can be surprising. In one recent study of three drugs used to treat severe heart rhythm abnormalities, for example, the researchers discovered that the death rates were *higher* among the patients randomly assigned to two of the three drugs than the death rate of patients randomly assigned to a placebo.[13] The third drug turned out not to be beneficial.

In other words, two of the three drugs were worse than nothing, and the third did no harm.

We need more studies that take a comparative scientific look at the actual results of various drugs. The same concept applies to tests. The Mayo Clinic, for example, recently conducted studies that showed one of the most commonly run tests for cancer detection is highly flawed and may be of little value. We need to apply scientific evaluation processes to our treatment choices, rather than rely too heavily on biased sales presentations.

COMPARATIVE ANALYSIS OF VARIOUS DRUGS AND TREATMENTS IS POSSIBLE AND DESIRABLE

Many HMOs now use a comparative pharmaceutical evaluation process that helps doctors select the right drugs.[14] In these HMOs, a committee of physicians and pharmacists develops a list of "best drugs" for use by the participating physicians. This list—usually referred to as the "formulary"—identifies drugs that are approved by the committee for specific purposes. When the drugs are identical, the lists typically favor lower-priced generic drugs over their higher-priced brand-name alternatives. They also favor—or at least include—lower-priced therapeutic equivalents when such alternatives exist.

Most independent-practice physicians do not receive that level of comparative information about their choice of prescriptions unless they take great pains to do the research themselves. For solo practitioners, research often isn't practical or feasible since they don't have the time or the resources. (The HMO teams usually include pharmacists—often Ph.D.-level pharmacologists—whose expertise in drug alternatives and composition exceeds that of most solo-practice physicians.)

In an organized care system, this research can be done through a central, dedicated staff and the information presented in a usable form to the participating care providers.

Similar approaches are needed for technology assessment and purchasing. The largest insurers and HMOs now perform fairly detailed technology assessments for their own use, but the benefits from those assessments typically do not extend to the community at large since they are typically not publicly distributed.

What is needed is a *Consumer Reports*-type program for health care technology that reviews alternative equipment and approaches in terms of cost, outcomes, durability, and ease of use. This information could be used by caregivers and care systems to determine whether or not to purchase technology and which technology to buy.

If reforms similar to those outlined in the last chapter of this book come into being—with teams of health care providers accountable for the costs and outcomes of care for the populations they serve—this type of information will become extremely useful.

JOINT PURCHASING OF LOW-VOLUME, HIGH-COST TECHNOLOGY

In an ideal arrangement, care teams could agree to band together in a purchasing pool to jointly purchase (or contract for) extremely expensive technology of proven merit whose use is limited enough that any given care system could not afford to be the exclusive owner. That type of joint-purchasing approach could bring technology costs down since the purchasing pool would insist on maxi-mum efficiency as part of the bid specification. This approach could avoid the technological redundancy we now have in this country. At the risk of repeating myself, there are now more MRIs in Phoenix alone than in all of Canada. That same comparison can be made for places like Minnesota, Los Angeles, and New York City—to give you some idea of how much technological redundancy this country now supports.

In Canada, they only have as much technology as the govern-ment's budget allows. In the United States, we have as much technology as can be justified based on its profitability. Neither country is doing the right thing—purchasing the amount of tech-nology that is actually needed. Both systems are seriously flawed: we overpurchase, and they ration. The answer, clearly, is in the middle—to purchase and use the right amount of technology.

Given the current incentives for our health care providers, our technological redundancy shouldn't surprise anyone.

Think about the financial incentives inherent in our current system: New technologies and new drugs generate profits for the people who manufacture and sell them. These new technologies also tend to generate profits for the health care professionals who use them.

In our society, health care buyers (insurers, employers, the government, individuals) almost always pay for new services on a lucrative fee-for-service basis, with the amount of payment not related in any way to the health care outcomes that result from the use of the technology. The result is an oversupply of technology and overall costs of care that continue to climb.

Almost without exception, the drug and technology-producing companies are publicly held, for-profit enterprises. They have to answer to stockholders, regulators, and bankers and have an obli-gation to generate profits. That's not an ignoble task, and I don't mean to be at all judgmental about either that objective or the way they go about it, particularly given the incentive that we, as a society, have set up for them.

I do, however, find it a bit easier to be judgmental about the caregivers who knowingly perform expensive services of little proven value simply to create personal revenue—and I am critical of providers who play on our basic ignorance and fear. Providers who suggest that we should spend billions of dollars on unnecessary tests because "otherwise we might miss something that could save your life" are deserving of our censure.

MAGICAL CURES

The issue of medical technology is a very sensitive area, emotionally and philosophically, for many people. Technology offers us the best chance we have for immortality. We, as a people, tend to want to live forever, and we want medical science to detect and cure whatever ails us. Our tolerance for "failure" by our medical system is very low. We want "magical" medical solutions to our every ache and pain. We particularly want our providers to save us from serious illness, and we want them to pull us back from the threshold of death.

We believe that medical miracles are our inalienable right as a people and that those miracles will be made possible by an ever-improving medical technology. That dream is continually reinforced by the fact that modern medical technology has, in fact, produced many of those miracles. Heart transplants symbolize exactly the type of care we want. The heart was long considered to be the core of our being, and now we can simply replace it when it fails us. That's powerful medicine, and we want more of it.

We also, however, want the costs of health care to go down. And we would like to provide health coverage and health care to the forty million Americans who are uninsured.

If we truly want to bring health care costs into line and extend coverage to all, we need to think hard about the process we've put in place to reward the purchase and the use of technology. We need to understand clearly what the trade-offs are relative to quality of care (and our dreams of immortality), and we need to understand where technology and drug development are now headed.

These issues are not simple. A recent study in California showed that when CPR was applied to patients who suffered cardiac arrests in the general medicine or surgical wards of a hospital, 58 percent of the patients were revived.[15] That's an encouraging number until you learn that only 5 percent of those patients ever recovered sufficiently to leave the hospital. For the rest of the patients, their revival triggered a "medical avalanche" of intensive (and extremely expensive) care and life-support systems, and the ultimate result was that most of the patients lived a short while longer on respirators and then died anyway.

What does this story tell us? In part, it raises the question of what caused 5 percent of the people to recover. To answer this, we need to know the characteristics of those people and how to make their number bigger. We also need to know if there was some way to tell that other patients had no chance of survival and that heroic care in their cases would have been totally futile.

We don't know that now. We should. That's clearly something we need to study, and then we need to make some choices about the extremely expensive application of technology where the only possible result is failure.

We probably have a lower tolerance for the natural aging and dying process than almost any culture, and we need to take that into account as we wrestle with the issues and incentives that relate to the health care technology industry in this country today.

The good news is that the answer is not the R word—rationing. Opponents of rational technology evaluation often invoke the specter of rationing to attack those who challenge the direction we've taken with medical technology in the United States.

Long before the R word is invoked, however, we should spend time and money on the E word—efficiency—and the O word— outcomes. We need to ask ourselves: Does this new technology or drug even work? Does it add value? Is there a less expensive alternative that creates the same—or better—outcomes?

The R word we need isn't "rationing," it's "rational decision making."

We need to use the drugs that work and the technology that actually improves results. If we make appropriate choices, we can both improve the quality of care and bring down its cost. At the same time, we need to deal with the fact that, although many new drugs and treatment approaches really do perform miracles, not all new drugs or technology approaches truly improve care. In too many cases, the increase in care quality from expensive technology and drug use is, in fact, zero.

Ask your doctor: Is there any evidence that routine fetal monitoring—comforting as it may be to the mother—actually improves birth outcomes? Is there any proof that ultrasound exams of all pregnant women—exciting as they may be to the new parents who get to take home Polaroid pictures of their unborn babies—have any measurable impact on successful pregnancies? In both cases, the jury is still out, yet the procedures are used in much of the country without question. We need to recognize that much of our system-wide investment in technology is unnecessary, wasteful, redundant, and driven by perverse incentives and that we do not, as a society, make very efficient use of much of our technological investment. We also need to recognize that there are few standards in place that can be used to measure the relative efficiency of competing drugs and technologies and that the current financial incentives of the provider are not based on choosing the most efficient approach to treatment.

We also need to recognize that drug and technology development is exploding and that the future costs and quality of health care will be directly affected by that explosion.

We need to move to an outcomes-focused care environment in which drug companies and technology manufacturers must sell their products to accountable teams of caregivers by proving their product's worth, not their product's marketability or ability to enhance a provider's revenue or profits.

If we move to an accountable health system, rational decision making will occur.

Insurers, Blues, and HMOs

The next question you might ask after reading about the negative impact of the perverse financial incentives we've created for our care providers is: "What role does the insurance industry play in the health care cost issue?"

The answer is that the insurance industry in this country is a major cause of our health care cost problems.

For starters, insurers pay care providers on a fee-for-service basis, thereby creating financial incentives that lead to high volumes of unnecessary care. To make matters worse, insurers traditionally have had very little involvement in the actual delivery of care, preferring, instead, to serve merely as unquestioning "conduits for cash" between the buyers of insurance and the caregivers.

To further compound the damage, insurers not only ignore the cost impact of their benefits on providers, they also tend to insulate the people they cover from the actual costs of specific incidents of care to the point where consumers in this country have little or no sense of the cost or relative value of the health care services they are using. (Consumers who are unaware of the costs or value of care cannot reward either efficiency or quality with their personal care decisions.)

If these negative impacts on U.S. health care were the only sins of the insurance industry in this country, they would be sufficient to justify rethinking the system. Sadly, however, the U.S. insurance industry has also failed in its traditional role as an efficient provider of insurance. Insurers have become risk-averse, making their money by avoiding high-risk populations and individuals. At the same time, due to the complexity of our multipayer insurance system, we have created an insurance-related administrative cost burden that dwarfs anything that exists anywhere else in the world. Government-run insurance programs like Medicare and Medicaid are prime culprits in this regard.

SINS OF THE INDUSTRY

The insurance industry in this country has traditionally

1. created perverse financial incentives for providers of care,

2. avoided any meaningful involvement in controlling the costs of care,

3. insulated the consumers of care from incentives or knowledge that would cause them to make value-based decisions about care,

4. created an insurance environment in which people are penalized (or excluded from coverage) for being sick, poor, or old,

5. created an administrative cost structure that is extremely wasteful and excessive.

By paying providers as individual businesses, rather than as teams of providers, the insurers have also perpetuated the current highly dysfunctional organization approach most commonly used in U.S. health care.

Perhaps the saddest fact of all is that while spending significantly more money on health care and health insurance per capita than any other nation in the world, we also have created a situation in which approximately forty million Americans have no insurance at all and perhaps a comparable number are significantly underinsured.[1]

Clearly there is room for improvement.

Let's take a closer look at each of these insurance industry shortcomings (in reverse order), starting with excessive administrative costs.

INSURANCE-RELATED ADMINISTRATIVE COSTS

How did we manage to create such a massive (and unique) administrative overburden to our health care system?

For starters, although many insurance companies have found health coverage to be unprofitable and no longer offer it, there are still nearly 1,500 different insurers writing health coverage in this country. There are also nearly 550 HMOs[2] and nearly 1,000 (PPOs)[3] and about eighty-six million persons are covered by self-insured plans, almost all of which hire third-party administrators (TPAs) to pay their claims.[4] No one knows how many TPAs exist in this country since most are unlicensed and there are no national regulations dealing with them, but there are at least a thousand.

Every single one of these more than four thousand insuring or administrative organizations has the potential to require health care providers and patients to use its own unique claims forms, membership data base, provider identification systems, and even cost-containment rules. A great many do so.

The cost of that much complexity is massive, particularly when you look at the extensive administrative infrastructures supported by various insurers, health plans, and administrators and at the direct cost impact of our insurance system on the care providers.

U.S. ADMINISTRATIVE COSTS DOUBLE CANADA'S

We really do not have exact numbers to tell us what the actual overall insurance-related costs are in the United States—down to the nearest $20 or $30 billion. We do, however, have some working estimates that give a good approximation.

Overall, the administrative burden associated with U.S. health care, including the insurance-related costs that are incurred in the providers' business offices, runs approximately in the range of 19 to 24 percent, according to the best available estimates.[5] This contrasts unfavorably with total administrative costs of only 8 to 11 percent for our neighbors to the north. Canada's administrative costs are lower primarily because Canada's single-payer system eliminates much of the direct insurance company administrative overhead and marketing expenses, as well as significantly reducing the insurance-related administrative costs incurred by providers of care.

In the United States, about half of the total insurance-related administrative expenses occur in the insurance companies themselves. The other half of these costs occur in the providers' offices in the form of billing clerks, bookkeepers, and other clerical staff. These costs exist because the providers are forced to comply with the various requirements of a multitude of U.S. insurers, government programs, and other payers.[6]

Interestingly, the single most burdensome source of wasteful and excessive administrative requirements for U.S. hospitals, doctors, and other care providers is the U.S. government itself through its Medicare and Medicaid systems. Although Medicare and Medicaid have relatively low administrative costs in their own offices for the claims they process, both of these federal programs have created massive levels of rules, regulations, and forms that have no parallel in Canada or in other national health systems. It's doubtful that the U.S.S.R., at its bureaucratic worst, imposed as heavy a paperwork burden on its care system as Medicare and Medicaid impose on ours. Our Medicare and Medicaid programs alone have created roughly twenty-six hundred pages of laws and regulations for health care providers in this country, not counting twenty-eight supplementary manuals.[7]

As an example, I am involved with a hospice program that is subject to Medicare regulations. The hospice nurses literally spend over half of their time doing government-required paperwork and less than half of their time caring for patients. They are working hard to get the paperwork time down to 30 percent over the next two years.

It's highly doubtful that anyone in Washington (or elsewhere) will ever need or use any of that paper. Compared to the Canadian system, it is a pure waste of health care resources. If the United States moved to a single-payer system but retained current Medicare and Medicaid administrative requirements as the way to administer a single-payer system, most of the provider-level administrative cost savings now found in the Canadian health care system would not be achievable in the United States.

Ask any U.S. hospital or nursing home administrator about the hidden costs associated with Medicare and Medicaid rules, regulations, and paperwork, and you'll receive an immediate education.

$100 BILLION COST DIFFERENCE FOR ADMINISTRATION

The best-known study of insurance-related administrative costs, done by Dr. Steffie Woolhandler and Dr. David Himmelstein of the Harvard Medical School,[8] stated that the potential administrative cost savings associated with a U.S. move to a Canadian-type single-payer system—assuming that the U.S. government would actually strip back both current Medicare and Medicaid administrative requirements to the bare-bones level of the Canadian national health system—would have been between $69 billion and $83.2 billion in 1987. Projecting costs forward at a reasonable rate (and ignoring any offsetting costs from possible increases in care volumes), that excess administrative cost could easily exceed $100 billion today.

That's a massive amount of money. It needs to be reduced. Administrative expenses in this country are clearly excessive.

COST BURDEN ON SMALL EMPLOYERS

In this country, the portion of our population who suffer most from high administrative costs are the small employers and individual purchasers of health coverage, who pay a highly disproportionate amount of their premiums for administrative costs. Larger employers can negotiate administrative cost charges. Smaller employers cannot, and because it truly does cost more per covered person to sell, rate, and bill a group of five persons compared to a group of five thousand persons, small employers pay through the nose. In fact, according to one estimate, the administrative costs charged by U.S. insurers in 1992 for groups with fewer than five employees ranged as high as 40 percent of premium payments,[9] with 20 percent reported as the minimum administrative charge level for that market.

If you combine that administrative cost percentage with the administrative costs that are created in the provider offices by our complex insurance process, that means that thirty to fifty cents out of every health premium dollar paid by individuals and small groups is spent merely to administer insurance plans for those buyers and as little as half of their premium is actually spent on care.

These numbers are so wasteful that they verge on abusive.

MARKETING-RELATED COSTS DWARF CANADIAN EQUIVALENTS

The single largest administrative burden that exists in this country that has no counterpart in Canada, Britain, and most other countries is marketing-related costs. In Canada, for example, coverage is universal and no one has to be prospected, convinced, or sold. Coverage is simply "issued." The administrative costs of issuing coverage is minuscule, even in the provinces that charge a small premium.

In this country, however, every single insurance contract is *sold* by someone, and there is a significant cost associated with the sales process. In some markets, that cost is unquestionably excessive. As an example, in this country, every small group has to be individually persuaded to purchase coverage and then must be individually underwritten (assessed for probable-risk levels), administered, billed, and renewed. Typically, in the small group and individual marketplace, the sales and renewal process require expensive face-to-face efforts by either agents or employees of the insurer.

The cumulative costs of these multiple face-to-face sales encounters are not cheap, particularly in the small group and individual markets, where the resultant sale may be for only one to five "covered lives."

A typical small-group sales commission in this country will, all by itself, exceed (as a percentage of premium) the entire administrative cost burden associated with a typical large group's coverage, including the costs of selling and renewing the large groups, sorting out their bills, monitoring the membership and eligibility rules, paying the claims, and generating utilization reports for the large buyer. Depending on the approach used by each insurer, those commissions can run from 5 to 30 percent of the premium for individual policies and from 2 to 20 percent for small groups.

In fact, the typical sales expense percentage in the small-group market in this country exceeds the entire administrative cost percentage associated with health care in Canada.

These sales and marketing costs are simply a fact of life in the current system. They will exist so long as our health coverage insurance distribution system requires this type of group-by-group sales effort. Our small-group sales approach in this country is a highly inefficient way of taking a product to market. We will not bring these costs into line until we implement the type of "small-group pooling" reform outlined in the final chapter.

If and when community-wide small group purchasing pools are created and properly administered, the total marketing and administrative costs associated with small-group products can be reduced by half, thus saving many billions of dollars.

Large employers, by contrast, usually have an insurance-related expense that runs between 7 and 15 percent, including any sales commissions that might be charged. It is clear that a focus of health care reform should be to bring small-group and individual-coverage administrative costs down to more reasonable levels.

HMO Administrative Burdens

Like insurers, many HMOs and PPOs are also guilty of participating in the insurance industry practices of creating their own claim forms, administrative procedures, and general administrative overhead. In fact, since HMOs and PPOs manage care and since many care management techniques involve extra paperwork or administrative procedures for the care providers, the administrative impact of some HMOs or PPOs on a care provider can actually exceed that of an insurer. The HMOs and PPOs, of course, justify that additional administrative burden by demonstrating that the total cost of care is reduced by their "administrative" cost-containment functions.

Not all HMOs are alike, however. Some resemble insurance companies by paying their care providers on a fee-for-service basis. These HMOs use rules and pricing arrangements to manage the costs of care and often have administrative cost levels that resemble fee-for-service insurers'. Other HMOs use a radically different structure and actually own the care system. In these HMOs, the care system and financing system are fully integrated.

The fully integrated HMO typically uses significantly less money for administration than either U.S. insurers or the Canadian single-payer system. Kaiser Permanente, for example, spends less than 5 percent of its revenue on administration,[10] indicating it is twice as efficient as the Canadian approach. In fact, if the Kaiser administrative numbers were attainable for all of U.S. health care, the resultant savings for the nation would be close to $150 billion.

The pure insurance-related administrative costs of HMOs vary widely, based largely on the HMO model, with administrative costs ranging from Kaiser's under 5 percent or so for a large, "vertically integrated" HMO that owns its own clinics and hospitals and employs its own medical and caregiver staff to the mid-teens for the HMOs that contract with large networks of independent physicians and hospitals and often pay them on some form of fee-for-service basis.

Even the least-efficient HMO models, however, achieve an administrative cost level that is better than the national average for all insurers, and those costs have been dropping as those HMOs have learned to be more efficient administrators over time.

ADMINISTRATIVE EFFICIENCIES

A reasonable question to ask at this point is, Do we have to move to a Canadian-style single-payer approach or to a Kaiser-like, vertically integrated care system to achieve administrative savings in this country, or are there other steps we can take that are faster and less radical and that still save money?

The answer is that major sales expense–related savings can be achieved by creating the small group cooperative purchasing arrangements outlined in Chapter 8. In addition, there is no reason why the HMOs, PPOs, TPAs, and insurers in this country cannot and should not work together to achieve most of the paperwork-related savings of the Canadian system by creating both a single, standardized claim form and a network of regional electronic (computer-to-computer) central clearinghouses to receive claims data from care providers. Under such a system, each care provider would be required to use just one claim form, rather than comply with hundreds of separate forms, and could send all of its claims electronically to a single source, rather than sorting claims and sending them to hundreds of different insurer addresses. The result of these simple and logical paperwork reforms—if the clearinghouse is run efficiently—would be to achieve two of the major efficiencies of the Canadian single-payer system: standardized forms and a single claims submission point.

The primary administrative cost advantages of the Canadian system for care providers are (1) a single claims form (compared to a great many claims forms used in this country) and (2) regionally centralized claims sites that receive all claims data from all providers in a given geographic region (compared to thousands of different addresses for thousands of different payers in this country).

The clearinghouse can electronically sort the claims and then send them electronically to each insurer for processing.

Both of these basic Canadian system advantages can be easily incorporated into the U.S. system, even before other levels of reform are achieved. As evidence, note that in Minnesota all insurers and HMOs have agreed to use a single claims form. A single electronic clearinghouse approach for claims is also being set up in Minnesota with the support of the federal government and our largest insurers and health plans.

It can be done.

How Do Consumers Benefit from Provider Savings?

The creation of common billing forms and central claims clearinghouses will not necessarily result in any savings to consumers relative to lower provider costs. The question to be resolved is, With millions of independent provider profit centers, how does society actually recover the cost savings (resulting from streamlined insurance administration) from the care providers?

It's easy to see how the insurers might reduce their rates to reflect their own administrative savings that can result from a single claims form and an electronic claims collection process, but how does one manage to win reduced fees from, for example, a small physician practice that has just been able to reduce its administrative staff by one billing clerk due to a system-wide administrative simplification? How does that reduction in the clinic's administrative staff affect the fee and cost of an office visit? Will that small medical group reduce any fees to reflect the lower cost of its insurance-related administration?

It probably won't. As health care is currently organized, the provider will simply realize the savings and keep the money.

Since roughly half of the excess administrative costs in this country are not in the insurance companies but in the providers' offices, according to the Harvard study, this is not an

> inconsequential question. It can probably only be answered in the context of the overall system-reform solutions proposed in the final chapter of this book since the current insurance payment system and independent provider organizational structure do not allow us to hold providers accountable for either efficiency or quality.

INAPPROPRIATE INSURANCE PRACTICES

In the best of all possible worlds, health insurance would be cheap and readily available to all. (In the very best of all possible worlds, it would be cheap, readily available, and a universal requirement for all citizens, so no one in this country would be uninsured.)

How does the current industry measure up against that goal?

About as badly as you would expect, given the economic incentives we have created for insurers in this country. Again, as with health care delivery, our insurance marketplace rewards outcomes we do not want. We have not rewarded our insurers for covering the broadest possible cross section of our population at the lowest possible cost. We have, instead, rewarded insurers for avoiding high-risk populations and for segregating the risk pool as much as possible in order to focus on profitable markets and market segments.

Again, as with physicians and other care providers, this doesn't mean that insurers are evil or that they are deliberately misperforming. They are simply playing the game according to the rules that we, as a society, have set for them. To change the outcome, we need to change the incentives and change the rules.

Before making some suggestions about the new product and the new rules, we need to take a look at the current environment to get a clearer understanding of the way things now work and the reasons for current insurer behavior.

RISK AVOIDANCE

As noted earlier, the traditional focus of U.S. insurance companies has not been on managing care but rather on avoiding "bad risks." Any good insurance underwriter can quickly rattle off a dozen or more techniques insurers use to help them avoid insuring sick or potentially sick people. Insurers have established health screening, demographic rating, experience-based rating, and dozens of other approaches that are intended to segment people into "insurable" and "uninsurable" classes. The net result is that (1) we don't use insurance dollars to make the health care delivery system more efficient, and (2) we have moved far from the socially beneficial insurance principle of spreading risk and health care expenses evenly across the broadest possible cross section of our society. We have settled, instead, on a system that rewards insurers for creating a massive, relatively risk-free cash flow, with the goal of diverting a portion of that cash flow into insurance company profits.

In the process, we've created an insurance system in which old, sick, and poor people too often either can't get coverage, can't retain coverage, or can't afford to purchase it.

That statement is not an exaggeration. It is clear to any reasonable observer that U.S. insurers try not to insure sick people. They charge much higher premiums to older people than to younger people, and they clearly discriminate on rates between the sexes.

Why do they do this?

Because that's what we, as a society, reward them for doing. In fact, we effectively force them to act in those socially harmful ways because of the rules of the current marketplace. Once any carrier can "risk skim," by enrolling only the healthiest portion of the population, all carriers are forced by resultant market and financial forces to do the same. Risk segregation policies, in fact, have become the only way insurers can make money. Let's examine why this is true.

In an ideal world, all insurers would offer their coverage to all potential purchasers without rejecting people for their current health status or prior use of health care. Also ideally, all insurers would offer consumers a single, affordable premium price that did not discriminate based on age, gender, or health status. In the current insurance marketplace, however, the insurers are allowed to reject the sick, increase premiums for the old, and discriminate against women. If any insurer in today's marketplace attempted to offer a community average rate while accepting all applicants, regardless of their health status, that insurer would quickly discover that its average rate would not be attractive to the young, healthy population who could purchase cheaper coverage from other insurers who offer price breaks to the young and healthy. The community average rate would, on the other hand, be very attractive to the older and sicker population that had been rejected or charged a high price by other carriers. The claims costs for those older, sicker people would immediately exceed the revenue generated by the "community average" premium. The insurers would lose money and, in time, would go out of business.

No insurer can afford to enroll populations whose claims expenses exceed the premiums they pay. Because of this, insurance in this country has become a game of skillful risk segmentation, with the goal of charging each risk segment an independently profitable rate. Insurers have developed great expertise in doing this and have adopted that approach as their appropriate functional role. Any carrier who doesn't play the game by the same risk-segregation rules will go broke.

As the president of one midlevel national insurance company told me, "We are totally opposed to anything resembling a community rate. Our goal is to rate each risk precisely, so each stands on its own merits. That's our expertise, and that's how we make our money."

That, of course, is bad public policy if you believe that an appropriate role for insurance in this country is to spread the risk of health care expenses equitably over the largest possible population, but it makes perfect economic sense for insurers in our current marketplace. An insurer that is too loose on health screening and too "imprecise" in the rates it charges will enroll disproportionate numbers of high-risk persons or groups who were already either rejected, "ridered" (the high-risk person has insurance with riders excepting coverage for certain stated conditions), or "rated up" by competitors. If that happens, claims expenses for that imprecise insurer will quickly exceed premium revenues and the company will go out of business.

That, clearly, is not an acceptable alternative for any sane insurer. No company can survive if its approach to the market guarantees that its expenses will exceed its revenues.

WE DON'T WANT STUPID INSURERS

To be fair, we can't expect insurers to be charities, and we really don't want them to be stupid. Insurance company stockholders definitely want the management of their companies to practice sound rating practices. Investors in insurance companies expect to be paid a fair dividend for their investment, and, as our insurance market now operates, they would be well advised to get rid of management staff who do not know how to rate "precisely."

More important, insurers also now have an ethical and financial obligation to their current customers to play by the rules of the "precisely rated" marketplace. Their current group customers and individually insured people deserve the security of knowing that the company that is selling them insurance is well run and financially stable and has sufficient revenue and adequate reserves to survive. No one wants to (or should) buy coverage from a company whose own survival is in question due to a consistent pattern of expenses that exceed income.

The truth is, we, as a society, have created a marketplace that offers incentives to our insurance systems that are, in their own right, as unfortunate as the fee-for-service incentives that our insurers, in turn, offer to our care providers. The particular dynamics and financial incentives of our competitive insurance

marketplace have forced insurers and HMOs into defensive underwriting practices. While these practices allow the insurers to
survive and even make some profits, they clearly do not work in
the best interest of bringing the maximum number of people
under the insurance umbrella. (Ironically, because of the particular competitive nature of our insurance marketplace, neither do
these unfortunate practices allow most insurers to make profits on
their health coverage much of the time, since the insurers compete
fiercely on price relative to the lower risk populations they all
attempt to serve.)

How did this particular set of market conditions come to be? A
brief review of the history of health coverage in this country
explains how the rules of the game were developed:

A HISTORY OF HEALTH INSURANCE

The original health insurance model in this country was the Blue
Cross system, originated by hospitals and schoolteachers in Dallas,
Texas, in 1929. The Blue Cross concept of guaranteeing a set
amount of hospital coverage for a flat, affordable monthly premium spread quickly throughout the country. By the mid-1930s,
Blue Cross plans were established in all states and covered millions
of people. All of these plans used the basic approach initiated by
the original Baylor plan, charging one rate for single persons and
another for families and using the same "community rate" for
everyone who applied, regardless of his or her health status.[11] The
community rate was based on the average cost of hospital care for
all Blue Cross members. It spread the costs of care equitably and
evenly across the entire covered population.

For years, the only underwriting requirement was the rule that
when a small employer offered Blue Cross coverage, everyone in
the group had to join. Blue Cross leadership didn't want just the
sick people in a given company to join. They wanted all employees, so they could maintain their philosophy of spreading the costs
of care over all members of the group.

Insurance companies, initially, had very little interest in the health coverage business. They preferred to insure more definable risks, like death and fire. But as the popularity of the Blue Cross approach grew—and as the physicians of America began to create equally popular Blue Shield plans that offered medical benefits side by side with the Blue Cross plan's hospital coverage—the insurers began to take notice.

One of the things that they noticed was the community rating practices of the Blues.

Insurance companies knew that risks varied. They understood underwriting. They knew that it wasn't profitable to sell fire insurance to the owner of a burning house, and they already knew that it wasn't good for their net profits to sell life insurance policies in the cancer ward of hospitals. They therefore concluded that there might be some valid-risk segregation judgments that could be applied profitably to health insurance as well.

They entered the new, Blue-dominated health coverage marketplace with the explicit goal of identifying and insuring only the lowest-risk groups and individuals. They accomplished this with several approaches, including offering lower rates to Blue Cross groups with younger people. They also introduced health screening to keep sicker people from being allowed to buy their coverage, and they began offering lower rates to the Blues' healthier groups and individuals.

As the insurers became increasingly successful in luring away the best, lowest-risk business from the overall Blue risk pool, the Blues inevitably found themselves insuring only the less healthy and more expensive segments of the population. As a result, Blue Cross community rates—based as they were on the average use of care by all Blue Cross–covered persons—were forced upward at an accelerating rate.

The process fed on itself, as the increasingly expensive Blue Cross community rate became less attractive to an increasing number of low-risk (and then medium-risk) groups, who then left the Blue Cross risk pool to purchase lower-cost coverage from the insurers.

SOME INSURERS STRONGLY SUPPORT PRICING
DISCRIMINATION BASED ON AGE, GENDER,
AND HEALTH STATUS

Some insurance industry people would argue strongly that the group-specific rating approaches are better for society than the old Blue Cross community rates. They argue that younger, healthier groups *should* pay less. They argue that, in fact, a return to community rating at this point in our history could force many younger individuals and groups (who pay less than the average or older payer under the current rating approaches) to drop coverage if they suddenly have to increase their payments to a community rate/average premium level.

The choices are between having each segment of the insurance marketplace "pay its own way" or spreading the costs of care across the entire population so that the young subsidize the old and the healthy subsidize the sick. The recommendations in the final chapter of this book lean toward spreading the risks of care, not segregating them.

The predatory, risk-segregating rating practices of the commercial insurance companies soon won the day. The Blues were forced out of the community rating business, except in those few states where the hospitals had strongly supported them with deep discounts that were sufficient to offset the costs of their high-risk pools.

For the most part, the Blues were reluctant and slow to join in the risk-segregation game, and, as a result, they often suffered major market-share losses before giving up on that particular point.

The insurance company-led movement away from community rating into various forms of risk-segregated rating approaches was a watershed event in the history of U.S. health funding. If the

Congress or the legislators at that time had the foresight to mandate that all carriers interested in writing health insurance coverage must use some appropriate variation of community rating, the current complex insurance rating and underwriting system in this country would never have come into existence.

The insurance industry and marketplace we face today is fully committed to risk segregation, in part, because that's the only way they know how to do business, and, in part, because risk segregation is now critical to their year-to-year financial survival. They are terrified to change. Insurers have tended to rigorously oppose any legislative attempts to significantly reform either underwriting or rating practices because they understand the current approach (and are fairly good at it) and because most reform proposals to date have been poorly conceived and incomplete in their scope.

Opposition to reform on the part of insurers frequently has resulted in proposing sham reform packages that actually preserve the status quo while purporting to accomplish reform.

RISK SEGREGATION IS BECOMING MORE SOPHISTICATED

At this time, while becoming much more sophisticated in their understanding of the public policy issues involved in health care reform, many insurers are increasing the intensity and scope of their risk-segregation practices.

Individual applicants for insurance coverage are screened with increasingly sophisticated techniques. Early versions of health screening only looked to see if the person actually applying for coverage had been treated for a high-cost condition in the recent past. Newer health screens sometimes reject people for coverage if their parents or other family members have an unattractive health history. For example, underwriters might reject an insurance applicant whose parents died young of heart disease or who has a family history of diabetes.

Individuals whose lifestyles might lead to high health costs—

such as sky divers or single men in their forties or fifties who might be gay (and, therefore, in a higher-risk category for AIDS)—may also find their applications for coverage either rejected or closely scrutinized.

SMALL GROUPS FACE UNDERWRITING BARRIERS

Small employer groups face many of the same health screening issues as individuals. Many insurance companies will refuse to insure an entire small group if one individual shows the potential to be a high-cost case. Other insurers will not insure the high-risk individual but will insure the rest of the group of people to be covered. This carving-out process can even include terminating employment for the high-risk person in some instances so that the employer can purchase health insurance for other employers at an affordable price. In other instances, a high-risk employee's particular health condition may be ridered.

Carriers also use "preexisting condition exclusion" provisions in their contracts to allow them to exclude benefits for any health condition that existed prior to the issuance of the insurance. (Preexisting condition exclusions usually are time-limited and disappear after a specified time period, usually ranging from six months to two years.)

To make matters even more difficult for the small-to-medium-sized employer, if one of his or her employees becomes seriously ill with a condition that requires ongoing expensive treatment, insurers in most states have the unilateral option of canceling coverage for the entire group or of giving the group such a huge rate increase that it either voluntarily cancels coverage or becomes profitable for the insurer based on the sheer size of the premium. Such rate increases, of 50 to 80 percent, for small groups are not anywhere as rare as they should be. (It's not unheard of for these rate increases to be given as midyear surprises—months before a group's expected annual renewal date—if the group seems to be particularly expensive for the insurer.)

It is true, in today's multicarrier, competitive marketplace, that a small group that receives a terrible rate increase can elect to shop for other coverage. Insurers, in fact, point out that possibility as justification for the existence of so many insurers. The unfortunate truth, however, is that other insurers are also going to be very reluctant to issue coverage to a known high-cost employer. For medium-sized groups, prospective insurers will insist on seeing utilization reports from the group's current insurer before issuing rates or coverage. For smaller groups, the prospective carrier will either health-screen all employees and their families or simply refuse to offer coverage if the group has either changed carriers several times over a few years or recently received a very high rate increase from a prior carrier. In each case, the insurers are looking to avoid having to insure costly cases.

Again, like the move from community rating to risk-segregated rating, this is a situation that feeds on itself. Once any segment of the insurer market practices these kinds of risk-skimming approaches, the rest of the market is forced to follow along or be left with the higher-cost, uninsurable portion of the business.

POOLED RISK APPROACHES FOR SMALL GROUPS

Over the years, a number of attempts have been made to create more "user-friendly" insurance products. Some of these attempts have been based on the concept of many small groups banding together to create large risk pools in order to somehow reduce costs and stabilize risks. For anyone who believes that either cost savings or reform can be accomplished by bringing large numbers of small groups together voluntarily into a single risk pool under the rules of today's marketplace, reading an explanation of that process is well worth your while.

One of the more highly publicized tragedies of the insurance industry was the bankruptcies of a number of Multiple Employer Trusts (METs) in the 1980s. These trusts were most often set up by various business associations or coalitions to offer affordable coverage to the small-group marketplace. They often were created with a commitment to use some user-friendly variation on community rating. They were often formed in response to various levels of insurance company risk-segregation and risk-specific pricing techniques in the small-group market. The founders of the trusts frequently created them with the express goal of offering coverage to all (or almost all) groups who applied.[12]

The people who created these trusts believed that large pools of small groups could, by sheer force of numbers, achieve the economies of scale, rate stability, and pricing advantages usually enjoyed only by much larger groups.

The actual results, however, on a smaller scale, far too often paralleled the historical Blue Cross risk-selection example discussed earlier.

These small-group pools might have succeeded, had they been the only insurers in the market. They, however, were not, and the U.S. insurance market is merciless in its quest for profitable risk segregation. Within a very few years, competing insurers will often lure the best-risk groups away from such voluntary small-group pools, leaving them with a deteriorated risk situation, increasing costs, and, ultimately, unaffordable rates. (Please see the following box on "Voluntary Market Small Group Pools" for an explanation of the process, if it isn't already clear.)

VOLUNTARY MARKET SMALL GROUP POOLS

Partly from either optimism or naïveté and partly from a desire to create sales by offering a very low rate, many organizations that created voluntary small group pools, or trusts, often based their initial prices on the assumption that they would be able to sell coverage to small groups, which, in the aggregate, would represent a reasonable and average (or better) spread of risk. Unless they applied the same health-screening techniques already used by the insurers in the marketplace, however, they, often, immediately attracted disproportionate numbers of smaller groups whose utilization characteristics (sick or older people) had already caused other carriers to either give them high rates or reject them altogether. Again, that only makes sense. The groups most likely to be shopping for coverage are the ones whose own rates have recently been significantly increased. Happy groups seldom shop.

This situation often isn't immediately apparent to the trusts or their customers, however, since the trusts also often managed to initially enroll a misleading number of healthy groups that were attracted by the idea of an affordable small-group pool and found the pool's initial rates to be very price-competitive. In fact, the creation of these multiple-employer pools was often hailed as a major success in their first few years of operation.

But over time, a clearer picture of the actual health-risk pool in each trust became evident. It sometimes took a couple of years for the real problems to appear since the small-employer pools also often experience another phenomenon that can serve to mask even very significant risk-pool problems for a while. As the pools quickly grow, they benefit from the "claims lag" phenomenon or, as it is known in the industry, the "Incurred But Not Reported" (IBNR) claims lag.[13] Typically, for purely logistical reasons, it takes about two months from the time that a group becomes insured until claims start appearing for its members. This is because the physicians and hospitals who treat them don't do over-night billing. In fact, it often takes a good while for the doctor or hospital to issue a bill, and it usually takes a bit longer for the patient who receives the bill to file the claim. The net result of these delays is that the first two or even three months of insurance for a group often represent almost pure income and minimal expense for the risk pool since the premium is being paid but the claims have yet to arrive at the insurer's mailbox.

Responsible insurers, naturally, create a reserve for these

claims because the insurers know that health care has been delivered, that the claims have, indeed, actually been incurred, and that the claim forms will soon arrive. They are not misled by the fact that the claim has yet to be either filed with the insurer or processed.

The multiple-employer trusts, nonetheless, have been known to understate significantly the size of this initial liability, particularly if their rating estimates were honestly (albeit, optimistically) based on the belief that they would enroll healthier groups than the risk pool they actually attracted. Therefore, they sometimes understated their first-year claims liability by as much as 20 percent by relying too heavily on cash flow indicators and not enough on actuarially based claims estimates.

This "masking" of the real cost of coverage can continue as long as the pool continues to grow and adds significant volumes of new business. When growth slows or stops, however, and when the actual annualized claims costs become painfully evident, a higher rate need for the trust's small-group pool too often becomes increasingly necessary. At that point, the pool managers have two choices: to follow insurance company risk-segregation practices by getting rid of the high-cost groups that are causing losses (by canceling them or bombing them with very high rates specific to their groups) or to increase the rates for all members of the pool to maintain the community rating concept.

If the latter approach is used, everyone's rates go up significantly and the community rate versus the experience rate skim cycle starts all over again: The better-risk groups quickly find themselves able to buy cheaper coverage elsewhere. The remaining members of the pool are, increasingly, the higher-risk members, and the cost of their premiums increases. As this happens, other lower-risk groups in the pool tend to find cheaper alternatives to these pools' rates elsewhere and the risk pool continues to shrink and to deteriorate.

Ultimately, if the small-group pool continues to use a community rating approach based on its own utilization, the pool will contain only a very small number of basically uninsurable groups. Then, to add injury to injury, any misjudgments that occurred earlier relative to underestimating the liability for unreported claims also come home to roost with a vengeance. The two or more months of claims-free income at the beginning of a group's coverage is usually almost exactly offset by two months or more of claims that continue to arrive for payment after the group has canceled coverage. As groups leave the risk pool, they take their premium payments elsewhere. The trust risk pool, however, continues to face the cost of claims that were incurred before each group's coverage was canceled, but which were reported to the trust after the cancellation. (It's not uncommon for claims to trickle in for six months to a year after a group has canceled coverage.)

If the rates for the groups that left the risk pool did not contain a sufficient rate factor for the IBNR reserve, the result can be a disaster for the last few remaining members of the pool. Pools have been known to be so underfunded that the final claims could not be paid at all, and some painful bankruptcies have occurred as a result.

I mention the problems with voluntary small-group risk pools to help you understand that there are powerful predatory forces at work in the current insurance marketplace that make significant voluntary reform by individual carriers or small buyer coalitions impossible, if not suicidal, and to point out that any future risk pools designed by the government will need to take the same factors into consideration or they, too, will fail.

This is not just theory for me. I had a personal experience, years ago, with a small-employer professional association that created a voluntary pool for its members. That pool failed miserably in its third year due to other insurers winning the good risks from the association.

I can also remember naïvely trying to liberalize small-group underwriting requirements for a very large carrier that I was then serving as vice president of marketing. We experienced roughly equivalent results, discovering quickly that you can't reform the risk-segregation marketplace one carrier at a time no matter how pure your intentions are.

In the second instance, after we agreed (as a community service) to help the small-group market by being a good bit softer than our competitors relative to health screening and other underwriting rules for a while, we quickly ended up with a disproportionate mess of very expensive, high-risk groups. The expenses for those groups significantly exceeded the premiums we were charging. When we looked into the results, we discovered that many of those disproportionately expensive groups had been carefully selected for us by various independent agents who were authorized to sell our coverage and who also represented other insurers. I called one of the worst offenders, took him to lunch, and asked him: "Why did you do that to us? Why did you give us your highest-risk groups?"

His answer made perfect sense, and I've never forgotten it. He said, "I gave you my worst groups because you were willing to take them and no one else would. I gave my best groups to another insurer because they paid a higher commission, and because they reward me if the groups I give them are profitable.

"I didn't feel guilty giving you the dogs because you were willing to take them and I figured you were big enough to know what you were doing. It didn't make sense to me, but gee, thanks. You made me a hero."

My company very quickly tightened up our underwriting rules, raised rates, increased our efforts to persuade low-risk groups to buy our coverage, and ultimately made the new risk pool marginally profitable, but not before losing a bundle of money and learning an important lesson about the predatory nature of the business.

There are roughly one million licensed insurance agents in this country who sell coverage.[14] Many of these agents represent several insurers, and they look for carriers who will take their highest-risk groups. Any carrier who wants high risk can have the losses that go with them.

As a result of this dynamic, the entire insurance marketplace usually health-screens individuals and small groups and applies restrictions and riders to coverage for people with current or potential health problems.

POOLING DOESN'T IMPROVE ANYONE'S HEALTH STATUS

One more key point about pooling small groups: It's important to realize that no magical advantage or improvement in overall health care utilization levels will occur simply because lots of small groups are combined (by one mechanism or another) into a larger group. I've frequently heard people say, "We could have small-group rates that look exactly like large-employer-group rates if we could just get a lot of small groups to band together." That's only true if the overall health characteristics of the small-group members look like the health characteristics of a typical large group.

If, however, the health status of the individual small groups who create the new "quasi-large group" was high risk before the small groups were combined into a larger pool, then the new overall pool will also be high risk and the rate needs will be proportionately high.

To put it simply, you don't improve the health status of ten thousand terminal cancer patients by combining them into a single pooled group. Insurance aggregations don't cure anyone of anything. Putting lots of high-risk people into a large group simply creates a large, high-risk group.

The only inherent advantage of this type of voluntary small-group pooling (under the rules of insurance competition in this country now) is that the rate needs of a larger aggregation of small groups can be more accurately predicted than the rate needs of any given small group, assuming that the pool is stable and that its constituent groups don't shop for coverage.

VOLUNTARY POOLING CAN REDUCE ADMINISTRATIVE COSTS—BUT NOT NECESSARILY

It is also possible, in some instances, to reduce administrative costs for small groups by lumping them into some kind of pool, but even that isn't necessarily true. In fact, when the coordination and planning costs associated with managing the typical aggregated risk pool are added to the functional costs that will logically continue to exist (relative to marketing, enrolling, billing, tracking utilization, and administering each small group), many small-group pooling projects actually end up adding net administrative expense, rather than reducing it.

Particularly in today's highly competitive, risk-segregated marketplace, about the only assured virtue of small-group pooling is some level of year-to-year rate stabilization for individual members of the pool. This is possible only if the pool itself has been carefully underwritten and if it can maintain consistent membership. The pool will have to insist on stabilizing for this to occur, for example, by requiring that pool members sign multiyear contracts. The truth is that only the type of community-wide, all-inclusive, mandatory-inclusion small-group pool described in the last chapter of this book offers any practical hope of reducing marketing expenses or administrative costs or of achieving rate stability. Any form of voluntary pooling in today's marketplace still faces all of the costs necessary to make the sale and to administer each group, as well as the additional costs needed to administer the pool. The marketing costs for voluntary pools will continue to be very high because these pools have to function in a highly competitive, dysfunctional, and predatory small-group marketplace.

AGE/SEX DISCRIMINATION

Risk segregation based on the health status of an individual or group isn't the only discriminatory approach used by today's health insurance industry. The insurance industry also discriminates based on the age and gender of the insured person. This means that women pay more for health coverage than men and that the rate difference between a twenty-year-old and a sixty-year-old can be upwards of $3,000 per year for individual coverage.

The gender-rating variance seems intuitively unfair since the major additional cost of care for women is related to childbearing and, in almost all instances, baby making involves a male as well. It's hard to justify, from a social policy perspective, why men shouldn't bear part of the cost of childbearing in their health premiums.

In the second situation, age rating, the rate difference can be so substantial that it can lead to hiring discrimination by employers, who can literally save thousands of dollars on health coverage for a single job by hiring a younger person, and to the lack of insurance for older, pre-Medicare people because coverage for someone their age is unaffordable. Increasingly, laid-off, early-retired, or self-employed older people below the age of Medicare eligibility (sixty-five) find they cannot afford private coverage.

Interestingly, the rate-segregation practices of the future may involve some additional issues that actually make better public policy sense. There is an increasing move, for example, to offer price breaks on insurance to nonsmokers since smoking has been proven to increase the health risks of users and since it is probably a little unfair for nonsmokers to put up with the environmental unpleasantness of smoking and then also pay for the additional health care expenses that the smokers require.

These types of price discriminations based on consumers' conscious lifestyle choices may make great sense as a way of encouraging healthier lifestyles. Rate differences based on smoking habits, for example, can be used to modify community rates.

Insurers Are Not Inherently Evil—They Are Reactionary

Again, at the risk of repeating myself, insurers do not segregate risk to be evil. Under the current market environment, they segregate risk to survive.

From the insurers' point of view, risk-pool segregation and the underwriting approaches mentioned above are crucial to their survival. Any player that softens its defenses in the current environment will quickly attract a disproportionate number of old or sick people who can't get coverage elsewhere at a comparable price, and that insurer will jeopardize its own financial viability.[15]

In that light, it's harder to criticize carriers for "unethical" behavior.

Our Approach to Insurance Is Dysfunctional

On the other hand, if you look at the insurance industry from the perspective of the small-group or individual buyer, or from the perspective of society in general, you see a very dysfunctional process that denies coverage to those who need it most. The hard reality is that the business goal of insurance companies is to collect more premium revenue than they have to pay out in claims and administrative costs. *We do not pay insurers to improve health care costs, efficiency, or quality, and we do not reward them for spreading risk across large populations!* We need to do these things if we expect a different approach on their part, and we need to protect insurers from their peers who would use inappropriate techniques to lure away their good risks.

The real irony of this situation, I often think, is that the insurers themselves usually do not end up making significant amounts of money from all of this risk segregation. Everyone is competing for those lowest-risk healthy groups and individuals, so those persons get rock-bottom rates from everyone. All insurers exclude high risks when they can. The net result is very small profits and, often, losses. Overall, the largest insurers have lost money on health care over the past several years. The net losses of the insurance industry on health care underwriting, for example, were almost $2 billion in 1986 and over $3.6 billion in both 1987 and 1988.[16] The net reserves of the Blue Cross system have been shrinking steadily for a decade in spite of massive premium increases. (See the box below for some thoughts about why insurers are losing money.)

WHY INSURERS LOSE MONEY IN SPITE OF THEIR BEST EFFORTS

There are three major reasons why the insurers lose money in spite of all efforts to enroll the best risks at profitable rates. These three reasons also explain why it is so difficult to evaluate the success of new products and approaches in the health care world in any time frame shorter than several years.

The first reason is that, although the insurers use various techniques to avoid enrolling high-risk people, the very best health screening only predicts future health care costs for about two years. After that, people's utilization "regresses to the mean" and their health care use starts looking like that of the rest of the population. So health screening has a time-limited benefit for insurers.

Insurers know that, in the aggregate, they can achieve lower first-year utilization by their new enrollees by roughly 25 to 40 percent by rejecting all applicants for coverage who are sick or have been sick. They also know that the utilization of the healthy people they do accept will look very average after only three years. This has been shown in study after study. The benefits of health screening to insurers are substantial, but very temporary.

This means that unless the insurers take additional and subsequent steps to get rid of the sickest people they insure as they become sick and identifiable (and some actually do that, as noted earlier), the expense level and rate need for the population covered is not manageable, over time, by risk-skimming practices alone.

The second major reason for insurance company losses is the increasing costs of health care. Insurers fairly often underestimate the increasing costs of care and lose money as a result. As noted above, insurers traditionally have had little or no impact on the actual utilization of care. Most insurers are only a conduit for money, receiving premiums, paying claims, and making or losing money based on the relative ratio between income and expenses. They have little or no impact on the actual cost, efficiency, or quality of care. When expenses exceed projections, insurers lose money. Since they have little impact on the efficiency of the utilization, this is not a rare occurrence.

The third major reason for insurance company losses is the highly competitive nature of the industry and the rate cycles that result from that competition. Insurers, in spite of their inefficiencies, are highly competitive with one another. That competition has traditionally manifested itself in periodic and highly predictable price wars.

Since the process is repetitious and cyclical, it doesn't have a beginning, as such. Therefore, I'll start the explanation, arbitrarily, at the "low-rate" point of the cycle. Periodically, due to highly competitive pricing strategies aimed at increasing market share, all carriers find themselves incurring financial losses. When that happens, the carriers become much less aggressive in their pricing and sales efforts. Their focus switches from market growth to financial survival. At that point, the insurers decide to raise rates for their current customers to levels that will allow the insurers to be profitable—even if those higher rates result in a loss of business. As the insurers raise their rates, that trend also takes pressure off the competitors' rates and, since everyone tends to lose money at about the same time, all carriers tend to raise rates simultaneously in order to regain profitability.

As rates go up, losses end and the carriers become increasingly profitable. This typically takes about eighteen to twenty-four months from the point in time when rates starting moving upwards.

When the carriers are fully profitable, they start thinking again about growth in market share. At this point, many carriers start reducing the size of their rate increases in order to grow in sales and market share. Intense pressure to reduce rates also comes from the buyers at this point since after a couple of years of higher-than-normal rate increases, the buyers begin to become somewhat militant about cost trends and begin to demand lower cost increases.

At this point in the cycle, insurers who do not bring down their cost trends find themselves losing business. In order for insurers to retain market share, all rate increases are forced down, and the cycle starts again.

As the insurer's rate-increase percentages shrink, and as health care costs continue to rise, insurers soon find themselves back in the unpleasant position of losing money. This also takes about eighteen to twenty-four months from the top of the profitability cycle. When those losses became painful enough, the industry again begins to "rate for recovery" and the upward cycle kicks back into gear. The buyers, having been lulled into a false sense of security by the prior year's temporary (and cyclical) reduction in trends, tend to tolerate an additional year or so of upward trend before again becoming militant.

The cycle roughly takes about six years to complete, with three profitable years for insurers typically followed by three loss years. Since it takes over a year to fully implement price increases across an insurer's total book of business, the price cycles are not exactly parallel with the profitability cycles. In fact, the rates the buyers see start going up about eighteen months before the carriers attain profitability, and they start going down about eighteen months before losses are incurred.

Because health care costs are increasing so rapidly, the loss portions of the cycle have been extremely expensive for insurers over the past decade, and the profitable portions have been less profitable.

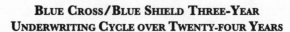

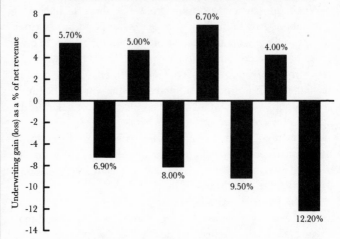

Source: Plan Financial Services, BC/BS Association; Milliman & Robertson, Inc., 1990

For the Blue Cross system, for example, the cycles have occurred at three-year intervals, without an exception, since 1965. Three years of profits have been followed by three years of losses. In the last up cycle, however, the Blues as a system added only 4 percent of net revenue to their reserves, and in the last down cycle, they lost over 12 percent of net revenue.[17]

So, in the aggregate, we have an insurance industry in this country that is extremely expensive but, at best, marginally profitable. We also have an industry that is unable to insure upwards of forty million Americans. Our insurance-related administrative costs are the highest in the world, and the relative percentage of money spent on care is the lowest.

Insurers regularly discriminate against people based on their age, sex, and health status, and insurers periodically engage in price wars that have little to do with health care costs but significantly cloud the health care cost issue. Insurers do all of this because that's what we, as a society, have inadvertently chosen to reward them for doing.

Having reviewed the insurers purely as insurers, let's return to their impact on the actual delivery of care.

CONSUMER INSULATION FROM THE COSTS OF THEIR CARE DECISIONS

Insurance industry apologists seeing this section heading will probably say, "What the heck is this—we get criticized for providing good coverage, too?"

The problem caused by the way insurance benefits are typically designed is this: Insured persons (consumers) are too often totally insulated from the cost and relative value of care, so they make inefficient and wasteful decisions about care.

In a "normal" economic environment, there are two parties: a buyer and a seller. The buyer evaluates the value of the goods or services he or she would like to purchase and identifies a price that he or she is willing to pay. The seller, at the same time, has also done an assessment of the work, raw materials, skill, time, and so forth that he or she has committed or will commit to the item or service to be purchased and has also determined a price.

In a normal economic setting, a number of negotiations and decisions now take place. If the price and conditions identified by both parties are the same, the deal is done. If, however, there is a disagreement, then either the deal is not done or some compromise is reached on either price or product.

Insured health care doesn't function like that at all. Rather than a two-party deal, with a buyer and a seller, we have a three-party deal, with a buyer, a seller, and a payer. The buyer is the patient. The seller is the health care provider. The payer is the insurer, the government, or the patient's employer.

It's easy to see how the introduction of a third party into the process entirely changes the equation. Think about the applicability of a parallel approach in other purchasing decisions. As Walter McClure likes to point out, consider how that same approach would work in letting people select their company car.

"Okay, Joe," the boss might say. "Here's the deal. You get a company car."

"What are the rules?" Joe might ask.

"It has to be a car," she responds. "You pick."

At that point, the likelihood of Joe picking a Yugo isn't high. Common sense might cause Joe to avoid a Corvette, but then again, maybe not. In any case, the car probably wouldn't be the car that Joe would have picked if the boss had said, "You pick the car—we'll pay half the cost."

Or if the boss had said, "You pick the car—we'll pay up to three hundred dollars a month as our share."

In health care, however, we tend to say the equivalent of "You pick the car—we pay." Although costs can easily vary by 50 percent or more between hospitals with equal services and results, employers tend to say, "Here's your health insurance—spend it where you will."

One has to believe that an insured, pregnant woman who knew that her maximum maternity benefit was $1,000 per day would lean toward a hospital whose daily rate was $1,000 or less, rather than select a hospital whose daily rate was $1,500 or more for the same services. That would particularly be true if the woman knew that the quality of care at the $1,000 hospital was as good as or better than the care at the $1,500 hospital.

We don't, however, factor either the cost or the value of care into the health coverage for most Americans. In today's health care marketplace, a pregnant woman in the example above wasn't even told that the obstetrician/hospital team she selected has a C-section rate that was twice as high as medical guidelines recommend or that her obstetrician had a very poor record for dealing with, and preventing, preterm births.

So our consumer makes health care choices with only an intuitive sense of value and almost no sense of cost. It's hard to get consumers to make cost-effective, value-based judgments about health care in that environment.

This is not an insignificant problem. There are wide differences in efficiency and quality between providers of care, but—as noted earlier—our current insurance system doesn't reward, recognize, or provide data to the buyers about either efficiency or quality. In fact, fee-for-service insurance approaches, in effect, actually penalize the hospital that only does necessary heart surgery and whose doctors prevent premature birth because, under fee-for-service medicine, it gets paid less money than the hospital across town that does those extra heart surgeries and cares for those preterm births.

CONSUMERS CAN BE UNREASONABLY DEMANDING

As a side effect of that insulation, consumers of health care can become unreasonably demanding. Since they don't know, and aren't directly affected by, the costs of care, and since they are not informed in any objective way about the value of care, they tend to ask for unnecessary or even futile care and can become upset when they don't get it.

As an example, a patient with a sore elbow may demand an MRI screening. A doctor whose focus is on appropriate care might say, "Well, we could do that, but I know what your problem is. An MRI scan will, at best, confirm my diagnosis, and it will make no difference in the treatment. There's a one in a thousand chance that you have some very strange and rare condition that can only be picked up by an MRI, but let's try this therapy first."

A typical patient reaction at this point, increasingly, is to say, "Listen. My friend Joe had the same problem, and he got an MRI. So did Uncle Henry, when his back hurt. I want one, too."

"Well," the doctor might say, "it won't change my treatment, and it will cost your insurer about seven hundred to nine hundred dollars for the test."

"Ah-ha!" the patient replies. "Just as I thought. You're trying to save money at my expense. Now I know I want that test."

And so it goes.

If that same patient were told, "Listen, the test isn't medically necessary, so I can't ask your insurance to pay for it, but if you really want it and will pay seven hundred dollars for it out of your own pocket, then I'll do it," then the patient's choice would become very interesting.

I was visiting with a doctor from the East Coast a while back who used that approach with a family whose grandmother was in the final days of her life. He advised the family that cancer had filled her body, that she was comatose and not likely to regain consciousness, and that she would die within the day.

The family huddled, then said to him, "We can't let Grandma go like this. Can't you hook her up to a respirator and some more tubes and keep her alive for a while longer?"

The doctor advised against that approach. The family insisted. After a brief discussion, they took a recess and agreed to meet again in half an hour to reach a conclusion.

"I was really depressed by the family's attitude," the doctor told me. "There was nothing we could do for Grandma except to painfully stretch out the dying process. Mentally, she was already gone."

Then, he had an idea. He returned to the family and said, "I will agree to do exactly as you've asked. I'll hook up the tubes, put her on the respirator, and do what I can to keep her breathing for a few more days . . . maybe even weeks.

"However," he added, "that care is not medically necessary. There is no hope of either recovery or improvement in her status. Therefore, neither I nor the hospital will be able to bill the insurance company. We need to make arrangements now, so at least the hospital will know which of you will be responsible for the bill if her estate doesn't cover it."

The family asked for a few minutes to talk the matter over. When they returned, they said, "We've been thinking about what you said. It would be cruel to Grandma to put her on that machine. Please make her passing as painless as you can."

That doctor clearly overstepped his bounds. He probably had

no authority to say that the insurer wouldn't pay because the care wasn't medically necessary. Please ignore that issue when you think about this story.

The point is, as soon as the family had the insulation of the insurance coverage stripped away from them, they had to look at the value of the care they were demanding and the cost of that care, and they made a different decision.

I do not and am not advocating that consumers should feel more financial pain for health care benefits. I strongly advocate comprehensive coverage for all citizens. Cost factors should be dealt with at a different level through a different process that puts the providers at risk for the cost and quality of the care. The point that I am making is this: In a three-corner deal, *someone* has to be concerned about value. If the patient is insulated by insurance from any sense of cost or value, then it must be the responsibility of the insurer to make sure that value enters the equation and that cost efficiency and quality are rewarded.

If neither the insurer/payer or the buyer/patient gets involved in these issues, then the seller/provider sets up all the rules. If we had a system like that, the result could be 30 to 50 percent more surgery than we need, defensive medicine, excessive technology, and rapidly escalating health care costs with no commensurate increase in the quality of care.

It could happen.

In fact, it has.

One final point about the issue of consumer insulation from the cost of care. Many of the more sophisticated buyers, who used to purchase full, comprehensive coverage, are beginning to insist on the use of at least nominal copayments in order to involve the patients more directly in the cost of care decisions. This can be a positive approach, particularly when done with the sophistication of a Honeywell Corporation, which developed a plan for their employees in which the copayments were designed by physicians to influence medical care, rather than designed by insurance underwriters simply to shift costs. (In the Honeywell approach, there are no copayments for chronic health care conditions, in which financial barriers to care can be counterproductive, but there are meaningful copayments for medical care relating to colds, flu, and other types of care, in which medical intervention, in most cases, offers little value.)

A more alarming trend is to significantly shift the cost of care to patients through the increasing use of very large front-end deductibles. In the small-group market, those deductibles are often set at $1,000 or more. That level of deductible might not be a hardship for a well-paid professional or executive, but it can be a major barrier to necessary primary care for people whose income is closer to the poverty line. A $1,000 deductible is the equivalent of no coverage at all for a single mother with small children and an income of $20,000 or less, for example. A $1,000 deductible provides protection for catastrophic care but offers no real coverage for basic primary care since the cost of that care will seldom exceed the deductible amount. Those children need coverage for primary care and preventive care more than they need catastrophic care.

The use of large deductibles, particularly for lower-income people, strips away far too much of the insulation from the consumer.

As noted above, if the patient is insulated from decisions about the cost and value of care by the insurer benefits, then the buyers and insurers need to get involved in that process.

INSURER FAILURE TO CONTROL CARE COSTS

As recently as a few months ago, I heard the president of a regional insurance company ask an audience of business leaders, "What do you want from us? We don't create health care costs. We just pay the claims."

That's the traditional position of U.S. insurers: "We don't create the costs—we just pay the claims." Twenty years ago, that was the topic of a speech frequently given by the head of our local Blue Cross plan: "We don't create your rates," he would tell audiences.

"You do. It's your use of care that creates claims. All we do is keep score and send you the bill." And he was right. That's exactly what both Blue Cross plans and insurers have traditionally done—keep score and send the bill.

More recently, some Blues plans and health insurers have begun to create a limited set of rules and regulations about health care delivery and to develop contracts with care providers that include those rules.

That's an inadequate response in the context of this health care cost crisis in which we find ourselves. Simply tinkering with the health care delivery system by attempting to impose some rules on an industry of independent, fee-driven care providers will not bring our costs into line or make health care delivery more efficient.

Instead, we need to bite the bullet and very directly couple the health care financing process with the care process, as other nations already have done. We need to recognize that the way we pay for care actually creates and drives the care system. The incentives we build into our payment process mold, structure, and sculpt our delivery process.

We need to recognize that it is financially and ethically irresponsible to waste money on redundant technology and health care profit-center "suboptimization," when we could be encouraging health care providers to work together as teams to improve quality and efficiency.

To allow the U.S. insurance industry to continue to ignore the quality or efficiency of the care it funds is both bad strategy and a waste of health care dollars. Any rational public policy for the 1990s ought to force insurers out of their "score-keeping" mode and into being active participants in improving the care process or out of the business altogether.

That brings us back to the first major shortcoming of the U.S. health insurance industry: its reliance on fee-for-service reimbursement as the only way of paying for care.

PERVERSE, COUNTERPRODUCTIVE, FEE-FOR-SERVICE PAYMENT APPROACHES

Earlier chapters about doctors, hospitals, and other care providers outlined some of the counterproductive impacts of fee-for-service reimbursement. Fee-for-service reimbursement is extremely clumsy as a tool for care system improvement, and it basically serves as an incentive plan for unnecessary services.

Let's first examine its clumsiness. In a fee-for-service payment approach, it's very difficult to shift the use of resources from undesirable to more desirable approaches. As an example, consider prenatal care. Everyone who has studied the issue knows that prenatal care is one of the best possible uses of the health care dollar. The savings that result from healthier mothers and healthier babies create a payback that is many times greater than the cost. Our fee-for-service payment system, however, tends to underpay for prenatal care, while, at the same time, it makes many millions of dollars available for neonatal care—care for the extremely premature and/or damaged babies.

Given the fact that we pay for process and not outcomes, we don't reward the caregivers who perform excellent prenatal care, and we throw riches at the providers who perform neonatal care.

Our neonatologists are the best in the world. They perform miracles, and they deserve to be extremely well paid for their skill and successes. But a more rational system would create a care environment in which we do such a good job on prenatal care that we need fewer miracles from neonatal care.

We can't create that type of system if we continue to rely on a nonsystem of independent providers whose financial needs are met on a piecework basis by fee-for-service reimbursement.

It's hard to reward a nonsystem for preventing premature births. Whom do you reward? The hospital? The obstetrician? Given the low occurrence of most serious conditions and treatments within any given physician's practice, it often isn't even statistically valid to hold an individual doctor accountable for many types of care outcomes.

It is very valid, however, both statistically and medically, to hold care systems accountable for outcomes when those systems represent teams of doctors using the same care protocols and providing care to a defined and measurable population.

Fee-for-service payments do not recognize teams. Fee-for-service payments do not recognize health care outcomes. Fee-for-service payments simply recognize units of work, whether or not they are appropriate or successful. It's a flawed way to create either quality or efficiency. It needs to be replaced.

We need to prepay our providers, as teams, for providing efficient, high-quality care whose outcomes are measurable and whose efficiency is real.

SELF-INSURANCE PROGRAMS ECHO INSURANCE APPROACHES

One last point about the way we purchase health care. Under a self-insurance plan, the employer takes on the direct financial risk for the costs of the employee benefit plan. The employers then, typically, hire someone else to pay the claims and administer the plan for them. The insurance companies who administer self-insurance plans for employers get to make their money by keeping part of the flow of cash that they administer, without being at risk in any way for the cost of care.

Just about every point made here about insurers applies equally to those many thousands of companies who self-insure. Self-insurers use fee-for-service approaches, pay for volumes of care rather than quality, insulate patients from the cost consequences of their actions, and create an administrative cost structure that is burdensome to the provider community. Self-insurers do not, typically, discriminate based on age, sex, or health status, although there have been a very few circumstances where they have taken steps that could be considered extremely discriminatory (such as capping coverage for AIDS victims at a very low level or using very long preexisting-condition exclusions that could result in people being uninsured when they very much need coverage).

Overall, however, the self-insured companies have simply

tended to mirror the dysfunctional practices and structure of the large insurers. That isn't entirely coincidental since almost all health insurers also serve as administrators for self-insured plans offered by their clients. Companies like Prudential, Ætna, and the Blues, all serve as self-insurance administrators. For many insurers, that represents the ultimate in the risk-avoidance goal mentioned earlier in this chapter.

Self-insurance administration can actually be wonderful business for the traditional insurers. If they are selected to administer self-insurance for an employer, they get to make money without having to insure anything. True, they lose the chance to make profits if utilization is significantly lower than the rates charged, but they also lose the risk of paying for unexpectedly costly care if utilization is significantly higher than expected because the employer has assumed that risk.

Insurers will often sell "reinsurance" to self-insured employers. Reinsurance, typically, provides coverage for catastrophic cases that might occur within a group. Reinsurance also can be purchased to provide coverage if the overall utilization of the group in any given year exceeds the projected cost level for the group by some predetermined percentage, usually 20 percent or more. In either case, the reinsurers' risk exposure is not very great and the premiums can be profitable for the insurers. The reinsurance market isn't all that competitive and has a high tolerance for insurer profits.

REFORM SELF-INSURANCE

There are a lot of reasons why self-insurance can be a good business decision for an employer. Cash flow is one of those reasons. A self-insured employer can hold his or her own cash reserves for future care and can profit from the investments of these reserves, rather than have an insurer hold those same reserves and keep the profit from that same investment.

But there are two important downsides to self-insurance in this country. One is that the same federal law that protects and allows for self-insurance (Employee Retirement Income Security Act—ERISA) also serves as the major stumbling block for health care reform in individual states. ERISA preempts all state laws regarding self-insurance, thereby removing eighty-six million self-insured people from state reform efforts.

The self-insured companies have good and valid reasons for wanting to maintain their ERISA preemption of state laws. The best is that without ERISA, employers who have employees in many states could end up being subjected to a helter-skelter of benefit laws in each of those many states.

The ERISA preemption issue will need to be resolved before significant reform can occur, however. For example, some modifications will be necessary to allow for meaningful state pilot programs.

The second major issue for self-insurers is the limitation that the use of ERISA now imposes on the ways self-insured companies can contract for care. In that regard, the ERISA preemption from state laws is a double-edged sword that can cut against the self-insured companies relative to their ability to control health care costs by putting providers at risk for the cost of care. While the self-insured companies are not subject to state insurance laws, they are prevented from entering into very desirable prepayment contracts with comprehensive networks of care providers because when such provider networks accept aggregate risk from the self-insured employer, that employer may have transferred part of the risk and is no longer self-insured. The companies may have, in effect, purchased "insurance" from the care providers. Equally important, the care providers themselves, by accepting risk as an aggregated system, may legally have become some form of insurer and could be subject to their state's laws governing either insurers or HMOs. As that happens, the benefits of ERISA could disappear.

It may well be that a significant ERISA reform that needs to occur is the extension of the ERISA blanket over those care providers who choose to contract on a prepaid basis with ERISA-protected self-insurers. That extension of the ERISA preemption would allow self-insurers to achieve the benefits of putting care providers at financial risk through prepayment approaches without giving up other ERISA protections. It makes sense as public policy because the basic liability for the coverage would stay with the employer, who would be able to negotiate a more rational and favorable deal with the care providers.

The right to enter into such relationships probably ought to be restricted to employers whose employee population is large enough to justify self-insurance and whose financial condition is solid enough to bear the risk.

If this particular reform cannot happen, then the dark side of ERISA may well be that the self-insured companies it protects will be condemned to continue using fee-for-service compensation as their payment approach when fee-for-service payment is obviously severely flawed.

OVERALL REFORM IS NEEDED

Overall, the insurance industry, like our health care providers, operates under economic incentives that work against efficient care and cost-effective administration. Reform is clearly needed to create a common set of incentives for insurers and caregivers that will result in an integrated approach to funding and care delivery, rather than the current counterproductive separation of funding and care. Reform for both is needed, and the reform is all of one piece. Reform of either insurance or care delivery alone will be doomed to fail.

Insurers, as they have traditionally functioned, add little or no value to either health care delivery or financing. They are risk-averse, expensive, and administratively wasteful, and they discriminate against the people who need them most.

They behave in these inappropriate ways because that is what the current insurance marketplace rewards them for doing. If we want to see a different insurance result, we will need to reward insurers for spreading risk, improving the cost and quality of care, and for creating the most administratively efficient linkages with care systems.

We will need to create marketplace rules that will prevent any segment of the insurance industry from prospering by risk skimming or by destroying another carrier's risk pool. Competition should be based on quality and efficiency, not risk-pool gamesmanship.

The reform proposals in the last chapter of this book explain how that type of system could be created. It is irresponsible of us to do less.

THE GOVERNMENT'S ROLE IN CREATING THIS MESS

The government of this country already has sufficient leverage as this nation's largest direct purchaser of health care services and insurance to substantially reform our health care delivery nonsystem.

Because we have not had anything remotely resembling a national health care strategy in this country, that immense leverage has gone unused. Rather than serving as an agent of improvement and reform, our government has, instead, been a passive purchaser of services and a major cause of our health care cost problems.

Before looking at the ways that the U.S. government exacerbates our health care cost problems, let's take a look at the immense health care purchasing power that our government already has.

If we assume that the total cost of health care in this country for 1993 will be $900 billion, then a reasonable estimate is that the government—in all of its various forms and programs—will directly pay about $374 billion, or 41.6 percent, of the total bill.[1]

Let's look at the component parts of that staggering $374 billion expense. Government payments through the Medicare program alone will total about $150 billion. Medicaid payments, including the portion paid by the states, will expend roughly another $157 billion.[2]

Most estimates of government spending on health care stop there, citing a total government expenditure of $307 billion. That, however, is not the whole story. Our tax dollars also pay for the health benefits of employees at many levels of government, including cities, counties, school systems, and state employees.

For the nearly nineteen million government employees[3] in this country, those benefits cost taxpayers roughly $67 billion[4] a year. (The Federal Employee Health Benefit Program alone cost more than $14.6 billion in 1992.[5])

This number does not include the $11.4 billion spent on the Veterans Administration hospital system,[6] several additional billions of dollars spent on the Indian health services[7] and other government public health programs. It also does not include the billions of dollars the government spends at the state and federal levels to fund various levels of health care research and health care education programs. (AIDS research alone costs the federal government about $1.2 billion a year.[8])

When you add the money spent for just the government-funded insurance benefit types of programs, the result is a staggering $374 billion in tax-generated dollars now spent by the government to pay for health insurance and health care services. That's an average of $1,399 per year for every child, woman, and man in this country.

By comparison, a rough estimate is that the British government will spend only $1,181 per individual to provide universal health care coverage in 1993. The German government will spend about $1,514 per individual and will also receive universal coverage for all citizens.[9]

The Japanese government will fund universal coverage with a total tax-supported expenditure of roughly $1,303 per individual.[10]

These numbers are estimates, but they are close enough to be used for comparative purposes.

In other words, our government *already* spends more tax money per citizen for health insurance than the average per capita payment ($1,332) of the governments in those other countries. The big difference—and it is a big difference—is that the governments of those countries use that money to achieve *universal health care coverage for all citizens*. We use it to fund coverage for less than a third of our citizens.

Frankly, it would be difficult to give our government a passing grade in health care resource use if we graded on a curve that included the rest of the industrialized world.

To make matters even worse, the growth in government spending on health care in this country now runs in excess of 11 percent. That compares, for example, with a British growth rate in health care spending from 1985 to 1990 of roughly 9 percent.[11]

WE PAY MORE TAXES FOR HEALTH COVERAGE THAN THE BRITISH, JAPANESE, AND GERMANS

One frequently cited argument against universal health care coverage in this country is that "our citizens would not stand for the tax burden that is charged against the people of Great Britain, Japan, and other countries to pay for their national health plans." The truth, however, is that the tax burden now charged Americans to pay for our current governmentally funded health care services is already running at 112 percent of the corresponding per capita tax on the citizens of Great Britain and Japan.

We, as citizens who pay taxes, already pay more than full price for universal coverage! The problem is that we don't get what we pay for.

Once you have absorbed the enormity of these numbers, the most logical question might well be, "If we can't seem to use that massive expenditure to buy universal coverage, is there any way we can use it to reform the current system?"

The answer, of course, is yes! The government could use the $374 billion it spends as a leverage tool to help reform our health care delivery system.

Without requiring any other reform, the government could say that, in three years, the only vendors able to sell coverage to the government (in all of its many forms) would be appropriately structured teams of health care providers created in accordance with the list of objectives outlined in the last chapter of this book. If the government chose to flex that particular muscle, the health care providers of this country would create those teams in ample time to meet any deadline. If a few large, private buyers voluntarily agreed to join that particular purchasing approach, the provider response would be both overwhelming and overnight. Health care providers are extremely market-sensitive, but the market has not understood how to use that leverage to best advantage.

The sad truth, however, is that the government, in spite of its existing massive purchasing power, has chosen to be a remarkably passive influence on both U.S. health care costs and efficiency. In fact, the government itself is clearly a major cause of the health care cost problems in this country.

This is due in part to a total lack of vision—or even interest—on the part of prior presidents about how health care might be reformed and an unwillingness on the part of the government to deal with the various powerful interest groups that have traditionally not supported any real system reform. The interest groups most affected by the government's use of its own purchasing power to achieve system reform include the government employees (and their unions), senior citizen groups (whose members might well resist being asked to receive benefits from accountable teams of providers), and the citizen/advocacy groups whose members worry about our poorest citizens being asked to receive care in a more cost-effective setting. These interest groups tend to be in accord with—and even more influential than—the health care providers whose strongest desire is also, invariably, to protect the status quo.

The truth is that these groups would probably accept reform that involves all citizens, but they may well not accept reform that focuses exclusively on the programs that cover them. That's understandable and even reasonable—but it is a shame because $374 billion in government spending is a lot of leverage to waste.

In what other ways is the government a part of the problem?

The government is also either the main problem or a key contributor to our health care cost dilemma in seven ways:

GOVERNMENT'S NEGATIVE IMPACTS

Fee-for-Service Reimbursements

For starters, the government is part of the problem because it—like the insurance companies in this country—insists on using fee-for-service payments as its method of reimbursing care providers.

As noted in the chapters of this book dealing with the health care providers, a fee-for-service reimbursement system that is not directly linked to health care outcomes or health status creates a constant financial incentive for the providers to perform unnecessary services and create unnecessary care complexity. An enlightened government could have chosen years ago to use and encourage a payment approach that rewarded efficiency and quality, rather than providing incentives for increasing volume and complexity.

To be fair, government has made a number of half-hearted attempts to use prepayment approaches for its Medicare and Medicaid programs. In these few programs, however, it has badly mismanaged the process relative to both administration and compensation.

What the government policymakers who continue to favor fee-for-service reimbursement seem not to understand is that fee-for-service payments—for all practical purposes—inefficiently, but effectively, structure the way the health care they pay for is delivered. This is a simple concept, once you recognize the extent to which health care is a business and understand the strong relationship between payment and provider behavior.

It really is not a difficult concept. Think about it for a minute. If there are three equally effective alternative ways for a physician (whose personal income is based on fees he or she is paid) to provide a service to a Medicare recipient—with one way generating a solid (and profitable) fee from Medicare, another generating a smaller, less profitable, fee, and the third care option generating no fee at all (but achieving an equal level of care for the patient)— almost all fee-for-service reimbursed providers of care will, of course, ignore the third (nonrevenue) alternative in favor of the two possibilities that generate revenue. The choice between these two alternatives is then very often heavily influenced by the relative profitability of each approach.

In other words, the actual delivery of care in this example is often structured *not* by the needs of the patient or by the relative efficiency of each possible approach but by the rigid definitions of care that are inherently locked into a fee-based system. Treatments that do not meet the definition of a fee-generating service simply are not done.

Periodic efforts to reform the fee system (like the recent attempt the federal government made to reapportion payment more fairly between primary-care and specialty-care providers) can make minor progress. That particular process met with great resistance by politically powerful specialty physicians, who gutted the reforms and significantly delayed implementation. As it exists, the result is a piecework, politically influenced unit-price fee schedule that still inappropriately and inefficiently structures the delivery of care.

DRGs Changed Incentives and Performance Followed

One interesting and partially successful government payment reform illustrates the impact of changing payment incentives very well: DRGs.

A few years ago, the federal government decided to stop paying for hospital care on a pure, unbundled, fee-for-service basis for Medicare enrollees. Instead, the hospitals were paid a single fee per hospital admission based on the patient's diagnosis. Those per-admission fees varied based on the patient's diagnosis, hence the term "DRGs" stands for diagnosis related groups. That single fee was the only payment the hospital received, regardless of the services the patient used or the length of his or her stay.

The system was and is far from perfect—and it continues to focus on one unit of care (hospitalization), rather than on the full range of care needed by any given patient—but it is a step in the right direction, and it has had a huge impact on the hospitals. Prior to DRGs, a great many hospitals routinely conducted an ongoing "revenue maximization" process for their Medicare patients, looking to bill Medicare for as many items and procedures as they possibly could for each patient they admitted.

Since the hospital fees paid by Medicare were deeply discounted, the goal of most hospitals was to offset at least partially the discounts by generating ever-increasing volumes of services for each Medicare patient. That strategy included keeping the patients in the hospital as long as possible because the last (unnecessary) days of a long hospital stay are the most profitable for a hospital.

Once DRGs went into effect, however, the hospitals changed their practices overnight. The committees that used to look for ways to maximize revenue became committees that sought to maximize efficiency.

Rather than ask staff if a given patient had received as many X-rays as might possibly be done, for example, the DRG-inspired question became: "Were all these X-rays needed?"

The doctors were brought into the process as part of the efficiency teams, and the net result was more efficient care, shorter lengths of stay, and greater cooperation between hospitals and caregivers in other, less acute, care settings such as nursing homes and home health programs.

The point of this example is not that DRGs are an unqualified success. (They are not—in part because they continue to focus on incidents of care.) The point is that *when the government changed the*

incentives, the providers immediately and effectively changed their practices.
The relationship between the incentives and the result was clear,
clean, and quick.

That's a lesson that the government needs to use as the best
advantage for all of us. In health care, as in other businesses, if you
want to predict the result of a payment process, just *look at the logical
outcomes of the incentives inherent in that process.* Discounts do *not* motivate quality or efficiency. They motivate volume, complexity, and
gamesmanship.

DRGs, on the other hand, rewarded efficiency in a particular
setting, so efficiency resulted in that setting.

That isn't magic. It's common sense.

Too Few Primary-Care Providers

The government also heavily subsidizes an education and training
program for health care professionals that produces too many
technology-dependent medical specialists and too few primary-
care physicians and caregivers.

In most other Western countries, primary-care physicians out-
number their specialty colleagues by a ratio of two to one. The
medical schools in those countries are geared to produce primary-
care doctors, who often have to practice in primary care for up to
ten years before even becoming eligible to enter subspecialty training.

We, on the other hand, have two or three specialists for every
primary-care doctor, and the ratio is getting worse. In 1992, only
14 percent of our medical residents chose primary care as their
field of practice.[12]

The health system reform issue that confronts us is what we, as
a nation, can do to create a medical education system that would
produce two or three times as many primary-care doctors and less
than half as many specialists and subspecialists?

To create a solution, we need to understand the causes of the
problem. As always, the issue boils down to financial incentives.

All first-year medical students know that subspecialty medicine pays a lot better than primary care. So long as we pay specialists and subspecialists on a fee-for-service basis (with fee schedules set up to reward handsomely procedure-oriented specialties for the volume and complexity of their services), the overwhelming financial incentives for debt-ridden medical students to choose these specialty areas will continue.

Again, the way to correct the problem is to change the incentives, not impose rules. Rules, as always, will only create dissension, conflict, and counterproductive behavior if they operate in opposition to incentives.

If, for example, we use a rules-based approach and try to ration the number of medical students who go into each specialty through some form of need-based quota system, the medical schools, the medical students, and the specialists will immediately actively resist the approach used—whatever it might be. Even if the schools were to agree with the quotas, the very process of determining which applicants would be chosen to receive wealth (by becoming subspecialists) would be complicated and difficult.

If, as an alternative, we change the basic incentives for all providers as outlined in the last chapter of this book by choosing to prepay our care providers as teams of caregivers, then these caregiver teams themselves will make their own decisions about the number of specialists and subspecialists they need. They will only want to pay for as many specialists as each health team really needs to achieve its targeted outcomes. If the teams are truly held accountable for the actual cost and outcomes of their care, then they will recruit the number of specialists necessary to accomplish those outcomes—but no more. Accountable teams of providers will not support redundant subspecialists or their ability to generate unnecessary services.

Once medical students realize that the care teams are not hiring or contracting with redundant subspecialists, the financial attractiveness of those specialties will disappear and the students will select specialties (like primary care) that will give them a better chance of being employed. In other words, if we create an environment of accountable care teams, the education system will self-correct to meet the needs of the new market and the result will very likely run close to a sixty-five to thirty-five primary-care to specialty-care ratio.

This will not only leave us with a current surplus of subspecialists, it will send a clear and immediate message back to this country's medical schools that subspecialty practices will at least temporarily be very scarce and probably less lucrative when they do become available.

Market-responsive medical schools will create programs to retrain redundant specialists as primary-care doctors and increase their focus on primary-care programs. The excess supply of our specialists could self-correct very quickly, with minimal need for government planning or intervention.

There are two clear roles for the government in this process, however. The first will be to create and support programs to retrain excess subspecialists, with the goal of teaching them to be good, effective primary-care physicians. (That process may take some retraining grants to help doctors make their mortgage payments during the training process.)

The second major government role will be subsidizing medical education so that our new primary-care doctors do not come out of medical school so deeply in debt that they need a large cash flow to survive. We are, again, almost unique among the major Western countries in requiring our physicians to pay for their education entirely on their own. You don't need to be a graduate economist to understand that the debt level of new U.S. doctors often causes them to make revenue-based practice choices that may not be in their own best interest, much less society's.

Other countries tend to subsidize these medical education expenses. We should do the same, even if it requires our tax money to do so. We ought to subsidize the education of at least primary-care doctors, nurse practitioners, midwives, and other front-line medical caregivers by lending them the basic education moneys and then recovering the loans by letting them—so long as they are primary-care practitioners—pay the loans back with some painless process (like allowing them to designate all tax dollars they pay beyond, say, 20 percent of their income as their loan payment).

That approach could create large numbers of primary caregivers at very little cost to the government, and it would keep them in primary care—at least until their debt was paid. From the government's perspective, it would be an investment, rather than an expense.

In any case, current government health education policy creates the very outcome we don't want—an oversupply of subspecialists and a shortage of primary caregivers. That policy is a large piece of our health care problem.

Science of the Nineties—Structure of the Forties

The science of medicine has changed drastically since the 1940s, but we continue to deliver health care in this country in the same organizational structure that we used fifty years ago, with separate profit centers and business units for every level of care and for every care site. It's hard to imagine a less efficient organizational approach or one that lends itself so poorly to accountability for the quality and outcomes of its care.

Rather than encourage providers to deliver care in the context of care systems, our government has continued to encourage non-systems and pay providers accordingly.

We need a government policy that recognizes that it is foolish and wasteful to think of health care as a series of unrelated, reactive care events. To improve the quality of health care in this country and to bring down its cost, U.S. health care policy needs to encourage, support, and even require a systems-based approach to delivering care. That means looking at health conditions, such as pregnancy, as being one part of a structured care process, rather than as individual and unrelated incidents of care.

A well-structured care process for pregnancy would start with prepregnancy education for the patient about reproduction (and contraception). It would include prepregnancy nutritional counseling and lifestyle education. Once a woman is pregnant, the process should include early screening for risks, followed by appropriate education and support for higher-risk mothers. The process should continue for all mothers through the pregnancy and delivery to include "best-practice" protocols dealing with C-sections and birth environments.

This "systems" approach to care really works.

The provable and practical result of this type of systematic approach for this country would be a 30 to 50 percent reduction in preterm births, a 30 to 50 percent reduction in the C-section rate, healthier mothers and babies, and a significantly less expensive birth process.

But that type of systematic, well-thought-out, carefully executed approach to care is not possible when each caregiver is a separate, unrelated profit center. It works best in the context of provider teams, in which the providers, as a true team, are accountable for the total maternal health of the mother and the well-being of the child.

Other examples abound. In the first chapter of this book I mentioned 185 consecutive deaths of comatose heart patients at a Rhode Island hospital. If a systems approach had been taken to that type of care, we wouldn't have an ambulance that had no systematic care relationship to the emergency room. We wouldn't have an emergency room with no systematic relationship to the intensive care unit. We wouldn't have cardiologists functioning as separate profit centers—with revenues unrelated to the care outcomes created in the hospital. Instead—as a number of more systems-based European countries have done—we might be injecting clot-dissolving drugs into the patient's heart in the home roughly ninety minutes earlier then patients typically receive such treatment initially in this country.

My own father died of a heart attack under exactly those circumstances, in an ambulance on the way to the hospital. The injection of a clot-dissolving drug into his heart in the home might have saved his life. We will never know, but we do know that a nonsystems approach to care was not sufficient for him.

But the government has taken no steps to encourage the growth of a systems approach to care. Common sense and medical science both tell us that any health care reform measures that are undertaken by states or by the federal government should be health systems-based. Any reform that simply fine-tunes the current nonsystem will not result in sufficient efficiencies to make the reform successful.

If the government decides to encourage the development of care systems—and if the American people (and the care purchasers) decide to hold caregivers accountable as teams for their quality and efficiency—we can make significant improvements in both areas.

Excessive Paperwork

Through its regulations for Medicare and Medicaid, the U.S. government creates the most overwhelming administrative burden for health care professionals of any government in the world. The rules and paperwork required to be a Medicare- or Medicaid-certified provider stretch the bounds of rationality and are expanding regularly. There are more than two thousand pages of laws and regulations for Medicare alone and twenty-six supplementary manuals.[13] These regulations add major costs to our care system.

For example, as noted elsewhere in this book, the amount of government-required paperwork to take care of home health patients in a Medicare-certified hospice takes nearly 50 percent of the time of the nurses who deliver the in-home care.

Why is this true? How did this happen?

The answer, in part, is that Medicare and Medicaid officials know that their fee-for-service payment system creates incentives for providers to deliver unnecessary care. Therefore, our government administrators want to see lots of paperwork that documents the necessity for that care.

Furthermore, because we don't have any system in place to measure and compare the outcomes of care for Medicare patients, our government has created massive sets of rules about the "process" of care in an attempt somehow to ensure the quality of the care being given. Since the government cannot, as data is now recorded, actually monitor the results of care, the approach it uses as a surrogate for quality measurement is to require very specific certification for various types of care, caregivers, and care sites and to create a large number of rules about the care process that often have little to do with either the efficiency or quality of actual care delivery.

Again, to be fair, in the current fee-for-service environment, where the outcomes of care are not measured and where each provider is a functional island, some of these care-process rules probably make some sense in spite of their costs because they do sometimes protect the patient.

But in a reformed health care delivery system in which providers are held accountable as teams for the total care of a patient— and where care outcomes and patient satisfaction are measured and publicly reported—many of these expensive regulations could and should be suspended. In fact, if that doesn't happen and the current oversight infrastructure stays fully in place, reform is likely to be severely handicapped.

The Canadian system achieves its administrative efficiencies, in large part, by *not* creating the kind of administrative burden that is standard operating procedure in this country for Medicare and Medicaid. Canadian health care providers could not afford the approach used by our government for its programs. We could double the Canadian health system's provider-related administrative costs overnight by imposing our regulations on their providers.

Some people contend that our Medicare and Medicaid systems are actually examples of administrative efficiency. Not true—although it is accurate that the costs of the pure, claims-paying insurance functions for Medicare and Medicaid are fairly low, comparing favorably with the Canadian system. Where our system creates great costs is in the provider rules and requirements that it imposes.

Any health care reform in this country will need to loosen the yoke of these unnecessary regulations, or success will be much more difficult.

No Sense of Long-term-Care/Acute-Care Linkages

The government has no sense of logical interrelationships between acute care and long-term care and treats them as two separate care systems from both reimbursement and programmatic perspectives. (Medicare pays for basic health care sources; only Medicaid pays for long-term care such as nursing homes and home health care.) This approach is arbitrary and wasteful, and it creates lower-quality care for the patients involved.

Long-term care constitutes nearly 19 percent of our nation's Medicaid expenses, representing a total cost to the country of $14.1 billion.[14] This portion of the government budget has been growing by 17 percent a year and shows no signs of slowing.[15]

Government expenses are only part of the long-term-care cost problem. Private citizens spent upwards of $18.3 billion last year in addition to the government's expenditures.[16] The growth rate of expenses in this area is particularly ominous when you realize that our country is aging and the number of people who will need nursing home care over the next decade could expand by as much as 43 percent.[17]

The logical question is, What, if anything, can be done about those expenses?

Government programs to date have attempted to control long-term-care costs in three ways: by holding down fees paid to providers, by tightening up on the definitions that determine how many people are eligible for long-term-care benefits, and by putting constraints on the number of nursing home facilities that can be built. Each of these approaches has had some mitigating impact on costs, but none of them deal with the real issue of how many people "need" these services.

In our society, in which health care is delivered in a nonsystem environment, the nursing facility also tends to be a business entity that stands alone, unrelated in any meaningful way to either the acute-care system or to alternative-treatment approaches for people who need long-term care. Payment is made for a particular basic unit of service, usually defined as a day of inpatient care, with some additional fees charged if a patient needs additional services. In a great many cases, this payment and care combination results in people being institutionalized who would much rather be cared for in their own homes.

A more reasonable, efficient, and patient-friendly approach, again, would be to pay a team of caregivers a prebudgeted amount of money for both acute care and long-term care, with the goal of providing the best possible care in the most appropriate setting. A truly reasonable approach would link that long-term-care payment with a comparable payment for the patient's acute medical care needs, with the goal of having the acute-care providers (doctors, hospitals) work on the same care team as the long-term-care providers (nursing homes, social workers, home health nurses) to create efficiency and quality care.

A number of experiments have already demonstrated that such integrated systems achieve greater efficiency, higher levels of patient satisfaction, and higher-quality care. The OnLoc program in San Francisco, for example, has been a success for a couple of decades and has shown that a linkage of this type can improve the quality of care and the quality of life for its patients. The four social HMO programs set up by the federal government on a pilot basis have also shown that costs are reduced and patient satisfaction enhanced with such an integrated approach. The National Chronic Care Consortium can point with pride to a dozen other settings in which similar efforts have achieved comparable results.

These programs have demonstrated that putting doctors and so-cial workers on the same care team—while revolutionary for both professions—benefits patients. The idea just plain makes sense.

There are three problems with that solution, however: (1) The federal bureaucracy is locked into perpetuating a permanent sepa-ration of acute- and long-term-care services by its own organiza-tion into separate Medicare and Medicaid entitlement programs, (2) politically, the government has not wanted to make waves with the senior population by moving it in any proactive way into prepaid care systems of any type, and (3) as the overall delivery of health care in this country is now structured, there are not enough organizations that are capable of becoming the type of account-able provider team that is necessary to make this integrated-care approach work. Attempts to integrate acute and long-term care have failed. They fail as a fee-for-service approach because—as always—the fees end up defining the care, and savings in one category of care cannot be used to create additional services in another care category.

The net result of our current nonintegrated care is a rapidly escalating long-term-care cost situation. A better solution is in plain sight but unused.

If, as was suggested in the preceding chapter, U.S. health care policy evolves in favor of accountable care teams, it will be a simple matter to extend that accountability to long-term care, with potential for major savings and significantly better care for the patients involved.

No Real Public Health Agenda

As Dr. Don Berwick, from the Harvard Community Health Plan, has pointed out, the major cause of health care costs is sickness. That's actually a pretty good point to keep in mind if we, as a country, intend to bring down health care costs.

If we take a look at the factors that either cause or exacerbate sickness in this country, a list of villains comes quickly to mind—

headed by the arch-villain, tobacco. Estimates vary widely, but conservative medical people believe that smoking is a major factor in cancer, heart disease, stroke, low-birth-weight babies—the list goes on and on.

The story has been repeatedly told about the medical school instructor in the 1920s who once convened his class specifically to examine a patient with a disease so rare that he said they might never see it in their entire medical careers. That disease was lung cancer.[18]

So what do we, as a society, do about this significant factor in health care quality and costs? Basically, nothing.

Although the government spends billions of dollars on public health programs, we really do not have a public health agenda in this country that effectively focuses our resources on such public programs as smoking cessation, childhood immunizations, and reducing the negative health impacts of pollution. Instead, we have a nonsystem of underfunded, unrelated partial programs whose relative effectiveness tends to be unmeasured and invisible and whose focus tends to be created by crisis, rather than by enlightened, systematic planning.

Given the fact that we don't hold any other part of our health care industry accountable for results, it's probably not at all surprising that we do not have an overall national program to improve the health status of Americans. That is a shame because anyone who steps back to take a process-oriented look at the situation would notice quickly not only that the largest cause of health care costs is, in fact, sickness but also that a great many of these sicknesses could be avoided, eliminated, or significantly mitigated if we dealt with them rationally and productively on both a policy and an operational level.

Let's think for a minute about the alternatives we have to doing nothing.

We could, if we really wanted to, create a national plan to eradicate smoking by the year 2000. This country has some of the most brilliant advertising people in the world. If we told them that they could spend $5.1 billion a year for five years[19] to run the most powerful antismoking campaign possible and if we funded that campaign with a $1-per-pack additional tax on cigarettes, how many smokers would quit during that time?

Probably a lot, particularly if we also created a wide availability of smoking-cessation programs at very affordable rates through our accountable teams of health care providers. And how many young people would decide not to smoke if they saw videotapes of dying cancer patients or ads showing the effect of tobacco on their breath and environment.

But we don't have a campaign like that any more than we have a clear campaign to end AIDS or a well-organized effort to make sure that all of our children are immunized against the basic childhood diseases.

Because we don't have a clear national public policy agenda, TB is reemerging as a scourge in some of our inner cities and other diseases that should have been eradicated are making a comeback.

We immunize only 64.9 percent of our children in this country. That compares to an immunization rate of 87.0 percent for Great Britain and 99.4 percent for Sweden.[20] In fact, we rank with third world countries on that basic measure of preventive health.

It's clear that we need a national public health agenda in this country that is targeted at some pretty basic performance levels. That type of agenda is almost impossible to achieve in our current health care nonsystem since it's impossible to tell which solo-practice physician is accountable for which patient relative to his or her overall health status. In the current system, doctors aren't accountable for the health status of the populations they serve, only for the specific incidents of care they get involved in.

This approach doesn't work if you're trying to create accountability for a high breast-cancer-detection rate. That level of accountability can only be created in the context of the accountable care teams described in the final chapter. Until such teams are created, we will have a hard time catching up even to Jamaica in immunizing our children.[21]

Hidden Taxes

To make matters even more complicated, we need to acknowledge that the government has chosen to fund its primary "entitlement" programs (Medicare and Medicaid) largely through a hidden tax that falls directly on all other purchasers of health care in this country. That hidden tax is the provider-fee "cost shift" that results from deep government price discounts for Medicare and Medicaid patients.

Discounts are not *cost* containment. They may provide short-term paper savings in the federal budgeting process, but they do not reduce overall health care costs in this country and they are not a very effective way of controlling even the government's health program cost trends. When Medicare totally froze medical fees a few years ago, physicians' bills increased by 16 percent and the total cost of medical care for Medicare patients went up by 23 percent during the freeze.[22]

When the government reduces the fees it pays for Medicare and Medicaid patients, care providers respond in several ways. They increase the number of services to "make it up in volume." They increase the complexity of services to generate higher, more profitable fees. They sometimes "game" the billing system by breaking a single service into multiple services for billing purposes. They attempt to improve the efficiency factors related to a given service to make discounted fees profitable.

Some providers even simply refuse to see Medicaid patients. (This is a real problem. It's hard, for example, for pregnant Medicaid beneficiaries to find an obstetrician who will treat them in a number of areas in this country.)

When all else fails, providers respond to Medicare and Medicaid fee-schedule reductions by charging other non-Medicare/Medicaid patients more money to make up for the government's shortfall payment. Insurers and private citizens who pay the higher fees that result from that "cost shifting" process are, in effect, subsidizing the government's discounts and paying a hidden tax that lets the government pretend the costs of Medicare and Medicaid are less than they really are.

Estimates of the cost-shifting impact of Medicare and Medicaid fees vary from provider to provider, but a common belief among providers is that cost shifts are roughly equal to 20 percent of current Medicare/Medicaid expenditures.

In other words, if you want to know the absolute full-cost impact of government-financed health care on the U.S. taxpayer, that invisible cost shift of roughly $61 billion should be added to the government spending equation—bringing the real cost of government health programs in this country up to $435 billion—or $1,629 per woman, man, and child. Again, if we average the British, Japanese, and German universal coverage systems at $1,332 per citizen, that comparison becomes truly depressing.

Cost shifting ought to be recognized for what it is—a hidden $60 billion tax that hides a significant portion of our government health care expenditures—as we consider future policy decisions.

The reasons for using a hidden tax are obvious. It doesn't receive much public attention, and, therefore, it generates little public opposition. It is a dedicated tax in that it stops entirely within the health care system. It doesn't face the significant political hurdles that an income tax, corporate tax, or property tax might meet if one of those tax sources were somehow designated as the way to bring Medicare and Medicaid payments up to full-cost levels.

As an invisible tax, it has traditionally inspired objections only from care providers, who bury it in other people's bills in any case. More recently, however, as major private-market health care purchasers have become more sophisticated about rising health care costs, we are beginning to see opposition to the cost-shift tax from businesses and other buyers.

It may make sense to continue using cost shifting as a way to fund government entitlement programs, but the days of that shift being invisible are numbered. The result should be a more responsible public policy debate on the issue and a better use of the approach in light of our overall health reform goals.

GOVERNMENT ATTEMPTS TO PREPAY MEDICARE

The largest single effort to use prepayment approaches for government programs started in 1985, when the government created a prepayment program that allowed HMOs to enroll Medicare enrollees in exchange for a monthly capitation payment.

That monthly capitation payment to the HMOs was set at 95 percent of the government's expected costs of caring for that same population on a fee-for-service basis. A formula was created to generate a county-by-county "average area per capita cost" number, which was further adjusted to reflect the age and gender of each Medicare recipient who enrolled in a participating county.

The results of that process were fascinating. In areas like Florida, where fee-for-service costs for Medicare are entirely out of control—ranging up to 60 percent beyond national cost averages on a per-person basis—the HMOs found a 5 percent discount to be a wonderfully good deal. As the fee-for-service costs in those areas have stayed high, the average capitation for Medicare recipients paid to HMO enrollees was $548 in 1993.[23]

By comparison, in areas like Minnesota, where the HMO market penetration is very high for both Medicare and under-sixty-five populations, the average monthly capitation paid to HMOs in 1992 was only $355—for providing comprehensive care to the same population that was being treated in Florida for $193 more per person per month.[24]

In Minnesota, due to years of HMO-driven managed competition focus, the total cost to Medicare for even non-HMO patients has been shrinking steadily relative to national averages. In fact, if the Minnesota cost trends for 1992 and 1993 were applied to the rest of the country, Medicare costs would have decreased nationally by $8 billion.

The government's response to those savings was to penalize the HMOs involved by significantly reducing the local rate of payment in comparison to national Medicare trends.

Without going into detail about the specifics, it can be said that the government designed capitation programs that directly penalized the health plans and communities that created efficiency and cost reductions and inappropriately rewarded communities whose costs and inefficiencies ranged far beyond the national norms.

Instead of supporting and nurturing a program that worked, the government chose to drive many prepaid health care providers back into a fee-for-service system that has clearly proven not to work so that the providers can bill the government on a fee-for-service basis in order to survive financially.

Let's look at the impact of that switch from a prepaid approach to a fee-for-service approach for one health system that made the switch. The "inpatient days per 1000 enrollees" ratio—a frequently used indicator of HMOs' relative effectiveness in controlling unnecessary hospital utilization—jumped from 2,066 days per thousand to 2,365 days per thousand for that health plan's Medicare patients in one year when that HMO shifted back from a prepaid program to a fee-for-service-based reimbursement. Medicare (and the taxpayers) paid for those additional days of hospitalization. When I asked that plan's CEO why the utilization jumped so much, he said, "Hey, we're not getting paid to control those costs anymore, so we can't afford to do it. We told them that would happen, but they did not care. They prefer a standard reimbursement, no matter what it costs them." Prepayment programs have been deliberately underpaid by the government, whose annual low-ball estimate of the upcoming year's average area per capita cost projection has become a running joke among HMOs.

$374 Billion Is a Lot of Leverage to Waste

Overall, it is a shame to let the $374 billion government purchasing leverage go to waste. We clearly need a uniform national health policy that affects all citizens equitably. In that context, the $374 billion can still be a massive leverage tool.

If the government really wants to see health care reform in this country, it needs to change the incentives for the caregivers and insurers. It needs to cut down on the red tape of Medicare and Medicaid and increase its role in monitoring and reporting care outcomes, and it needs to create a real public health agenda and then implement it successfully.

Each of these approaches will be much more successful if accountable teams of health care providers are used. For that reason, the government should do whatever it can to make such teams possible and then successful.

———■———

Chapter 7

CURRENT REFORM PROPOSALS AND OPTIONS

The key to reforming the American health care delivery system will be to align fully the health and cost objectives of the American people with the financial incentives and rewards that we offer to our health care providers and insurers.

If we assume that these objectives are high-quality, continuously improving, appropriately motivated health care that is affordable, efficient, accessible, and conveniently available—and if we assume that universal coverage for all Americans is also a reasonable objective for health care reform—then common sense tells us that we should measure each of the various health care reform proposals in terms of these objectives. These proposals have varied significantly, from a slight modification of the current nonsystem to a major restructuring of our health care delivery and financing approaches.

Some of the current proposals for health care reform do little more than fine-tune the current system and are therefore doomed to failure. Others deal directly with the underlying financial and structural issues facing health care and are more likely to be successful.

Let's look at each of the major options before outlining the best approach available.

CONTINUATION OF FEE-FOR-SERVICE STATUS QUO

Due to the complexity and political volatility of health care reform, it is possible that the final result of the current reform attempts will be a deadlock that, in effect, continues the status quo. But, since it is the status quo that is producing the very costs and results that the vast majority of the population finds unacceptable, the actual result would probably be a status quo with some very significant regulations added.

If other reforms fail, it's easy to predict that the government would probably attempt to save face and ingratiate itself with the populace by imposing some forms of fairly punitive and rigorous price and fee regulations on the current provider system. In addition, the politically acceptable approach might be to impose a number of "rules" relative to the actual delivery of care. In other words, a policy stalemate that results in the continuation of the current fee-for-service nonsystematic approach to health care will actually lead us to a health care world of regulations and rules that are at odds with the financial incentives of the system. In that heavily regulated fee-for-service environment, externally imposed rules about care utilization will do daily battle with the providers' own financial incentives and personal best interests. If that world occurs, then—as usual—the incentives will, at least initially, win because anyone smart enough to earn either an MHA (master's degree in hospital administration) or a medical degree is smart enough to generate high volumes of services and revenue by going around the rules. Read Chapter 2; it's easy.

Years ago, when Medicare had just sent out another set of payment rules to hospitals, I had a conversation with a hospital's chief financial officer about the impact of those rules on his hospital.

"They'll be a pain," he said, "but we'll get around them. We can beat any set of rules in less than a year—unless the rules are complicated. Then we can beat them in six months."

There may have been a hint of bravado in his statement, but there's an underlying truth to the concept that when rules clash with incentives, the incentives tend to win out. Creativity lines up on the side of the incentives.

It isn't easy to overcome incentives with rules. In order for a purely rules-based U.S. health care cost-containment approach to work, the rules would need to be pervasive, consistent, complex, highly sophisticated, very bureaucratic, and rigidly enforced by large numbers of highly skilled technicians—in other words, exactly the kind of system that lends itself to diagnostic and billing gamesmanship and to a counterproductive use of resources. That rules-driven approach is, in fact, basically the system that has already failed to keep costs in line for Medicare and Medicaid.

What is really sad is that in a rules-based cost-control approach, providers will focus their creativity on beating the rules in their own financial self-interest instead of focusing on creating an efficient and continuously improving health care system.

Furthermore, rules tend to destroy other innovation that can result in improvements in either quality or efficiency because rules tend to perpetuate a system as it exists at a given point in time. Rigidly enforced rules do not create an environment in which a system is encouraged, motivated, or even allowed to continuously improve its performance.

We will not move to the next level of more sophisticated and less costly care-site approaches under a rules-based system because the rules will lock the current system firmly into place.

A rules-based approach in a fee-for-service context cannot do the job we need to have done. The task would be immense. In addition to rules about the actual delivery of care, we would need to have rigidly enforced rules about how the billing for that care is done. The government would need to establish detailed unit prices for all care. The government would also need to figure out a way to ration the highest-cost, highest-tech care at a level the nation could afford since the specialty providers' revenue opportunities under a fee-for-service system would still cause providers to increase those costs at an otherwise unaffordable rate.

Rationing, in this country, would not be easy. High-tech care rationing in the United States would require Solomon's wisdom on the part of government and a sea change in expectations about health care on the part of the U.S. public. It's possible that we may acquire both the wisdom and the public will to create a workable, ethics-based rationing approach to high-tech care in this country, but it's hard to imagine. It is far easier to imagine a media parade of heartbreaking stories about patient tragedies in cases in which the government's rationing rules have caused care to be denied, with a resultant public outcry and subsequent political circuses.

In any environment managed by rules and rationing there's bound to be a public backlash against caregivers and government officials. The public and media will seek villains and scapegoats for health care costs and for the nonperformance of a regulated system and will find them at random points within the government and the care system. At that point, they will seek public punishment for the culprits.

In other words, continuation of the present fee-for-service paradigm for health care reimbursement—with the financial incentives of the providers permanently out of alignment with the health care objectives of the consumers—will be unproductive and probably fairly unpleasant.

ALTERNATE APPROACHES IN OTHER COUNTRIES

Other nations have avoided the battle between incentives and cost controls very nicely by moving away from fee-for-service care.

Great Britain
In Great Britain, the primary-care doctors are paid a flat

monthly fee for each patient who chooses to join the doctors "panel." Doctors compete with each other to make sure that their panels of patients are full by delivering care that the patients find satisfactory.

In other words, the British use a prepaid managed competition model for their primary-care doctors. They have eliminated the perverse incentives that come from fee-for-service payments.

The primary-care system is extremely popular with the British people, who would probably revolt if the government attempted to change that particular managed competition approach to primary care. Their system of capitated primary-care doctors who compete for patients creates responsive doctors whose primary focus is the patient's needs. That approach only applies to primary care, however.

At the specialty-care level, the British have adopted a less popular budget-controlled process. They very sensibly limit the number of doctors who can go into the medical specialties, and they put those doctors on salary.

The British government also owns the high-tech equipment, as well as almost all of the hospitals in which it is used.

By owning the high-tech and specialty-care systems, the British can control costs very directly by simply setting budgets for those levels of care and then allocating only the budgeted amount of funds to those institutions and programs. The high-tech and specialty providers of care help develop those budgets, based on the health needs of the populations they serve and on the availability of government money.

For the government-owned hospitals and government-employed medical specialists, those governmental budgets dictate salaries, operating revenue, capital investments, hiring practices, and the resource availability of high-tech/specialty care.

Once the budgets are in place, the care providers simply treat as many patients as they can with the resources available. This results in long wait times for many procedures that are quickly treated in this country (hip replacements and bypass surgery, for example) but also in a big reduction in unnecessary care and redundant technology.

Canada

With one important exception, the Canadian system is very similar to the British system. As in Great Britain, primary-care providers function as independent businesses and high-tech and hospital care is owned (or fully budget controlled) by the government.

The major difference between the two systems is that the primary-care doctors in Canada are paid on a fee-for-service basis, in contrast to the capitated approach used in Great Britain. The fee-for-service incentives in the Canadian primary-care system have made it the second most expensive care in the world—after the United States. In fact, the Canadian cost trends equal or exceed the cost trends for U.S. primary care. Canada's primary-care costs are lower than those in the United States only because the fee schedules used by the Canadian government are lower than ours, but the gap is narrowing.

Like Great Britain, Canada controls high-tech and specialty care through budgets, not fees. The Canadian health system decides how many MRIs will be purchased for a given region of Canada, and that decision is made based on the medical need and the availability of government money.

In the United States, these decisions are made by independent providers, and the potential profitability of the MRI is more of a driving factor than the medical need.

Germany

In Germany, the approach used is basically another version of managed competition, with vertically integrated care systems (doctors and hospitals functioning as a team) enrolling "members" and providing them with comprehensive care for a fixed price.

The German government controls the overall cost of care by regulating the revenue that those care systems can generate. The systems have to operate within the constraints of those revenue gaps, and they make their internal cost decisions accordingly.

Only in the United States do we have nonmanaged competition coupled with the perverse incentives of fee-for-service payment applied to all levels of care, from primary care through the highest-cost, technology-based subspecialty care.

Any health care reform in the United States that leaves that structure and those incentives in place will have to overcome them with a medical police state.

The good news is that no one is currently expecting the status quo to continue to that point. The chances of more progressive reform seem to be good as this is being written.

CANADIAN-STYLE SINGLE-PAYER SOLUTION

A number of health care activists have suggested that the simple solution to our health care cost problems might be to borrow the program used by our Canadian neighbors, a single-payer system in which the government is the sole payer of care and all citizens are issued coverage by the government. That system has some advantages. Converting the U.S. health care financing system to the Canadian single-payer system, would offer some hope of reducing the current high level of U.S. health care's finance-related administrative costs. As noted earlier, health care administration costs in Canada run far below those of the U.S. multipayer financing system. Under a Canadian-style system, rather than having to comply with the various billing and reporting approaches now used by fifteen hundred insurance companies, 550 HMOs, one thousand PPOs, a myriad of TPAs, and the various programs of the U.S. government, our health care providers could use a single claim form and send it to a single-payer source. This approach would clearly alleviate some of the administrative expenses U.S. caregivers now suffer.

But as was also pointed out earlier, if we were to create a U.S. version of the Canadian system by simply extending the current rules and regulations for either Medicare and Medicaid to all U.S. care, we would see very little positive impact on the insurance-related administrative burden for care providers.

In fact, those costs would be a multiple of the Canadian costs, because the Canadian government imposes a much lighter administrative burden on care providers than the U.S. government does. In Canada, the care provider performs a service and then merely submits a simple claim form to the government. That claim is just as simply paid by the regional government administrator according to a government fee schedule. Claims receive little or no review for either appropriateness or accuracy, and few, if any, questions are asked. There are very few rules requiring, for example, that clinic doors have to be forty-two inches wide or that only certified technicians can file certain records. In this country, the Medicare and Medicaid processes require much more information, cost justification, care detail, and compliance with extensive site-specific rules and regulations about the settings in which care can be delivered.

Let's be realistic. The likelihood of our current government bureaucracy peacefully giving up the massive set of rules and regulations of our government programs in order to achieve a Canadian level of payment simplicity is not very high.

To be fair to our government officials, using a simple, Canadian-style, highly trusting, nonjudgmental claims payment process might not be the smartest move we could make. It's reasonable to ask whether or not the trusting simplicity of the Canadian system might not be much abused in this country, particularly if it is applied to subspecialty, high-tech care. We've already had a sufficient number of billing scandals and proven abuse of the current U.S. billing process to give us reason to believe that this country might require a more sophisticated (and more expensive) billing and claims process than the Canadians now use. That additional complexity would, of course, erode a substantial piece of the administrative savings we might achieve.

Many Canadian health planners freely admit that their system is also flawed in its dependence on fee-for-service billing as its payment approach for primary care. As noted earlier, costs in care categories paid on that basis are going up as fast or faster than comparable costs in the United States.

Canada's Hospital and Specialist Budgets Are the Secret of Success

Perhaps the most important point to think about in considering an adoption of the Canadian care approach in this country is this: How would we transplant to the United States the key element that actually makes their plan work—absolute and direct budget control over all U.S. hospitals and specialty-care providers? Anyone who has looked at their system knows that the major reason for lower health care costs in Canada is *not* replacement of the insurance companies with a government single payer. The savings that result from single-payer status only make up about 10 percent of the cost difference between the countries. The major difference between their cost structure and ours—and the one most difficult for the United States to emulate—is that in Canada the areas of the highest potential for unnecessary expense (hospital, high-tech, and subspecialty care) are basically "owned" by the government. They are not independent fee-for-service providers of care. They receive a flat, prebudgeted payment from the government as their sole source of revenue.

This is a critical point to understand! The government in Canada can control costs directly by controlling its budgets. It does not use an indirect fee-setting control for its hospital and high-tech care. It saves money by deciding in advance how much care will be delivered. And if, for example, the Canadian government can't afford an MRI, it simply doesn't buy one or make it available.

We could not achieve the cost savings of the Canadian system by simply moving the single-payer approach south and applying it to all caregivers because in the United States private enterprise owns the MRIs and almost all the rest of the high-cost, high-tech specialty-care delivery system and the use of that equipment is paid for by U.S. insurers and the government on a fee-for-service basis. That's very different from the Canadian structure. I've yet to hear a proponent of a Canadian-style single-payer approach deal with that critical issue: How can we achieve that type of budget control over hospital, specialty, and high-tech care through a mechanism as clumsy as fee-for-service payment?

If we want the Canadian system to work in this country, we need to use the actual Canadian system. That raises some interesting questions. Would the U.S. government buy all American hospitals and specialty- and high-tech care sites in order to create a Canadian-type single-payer system? Would the government nationalize high-tech care? Would state or federal government create some sort of government agency to determine the annual budget for the Mayo Clinic, the Geisinger Medical Center in Danville, Pennsylvania, and the Carle Clinic in Urbana, Illinois? And even if some budgeting approach could be created for our great national clinics, how would we create separate taxpayer-supported budgets for each local hospital and subspecialty group? What would that cost? Could it even be done? Who would make what decisions? How and when? These are not irrelevant questions. If we can't answer them, we can't import the Canadian system because that is exactly what they do in Canada, and that approach is central to their success. If we skip that key part of the process, we will be deluding ourselves.

For the sake of argument, let's say we decide not to import the province-by-province and hospital-by-hospital budget approach of the Canadian system and decide instead to import just the single-payer insurance administration portion of the approach. If we do that, we need to break new ground and figure out how to modify the Canadian approach to pay the U.S. providers whose costs would be directly controlled in Canada by budget. The question is, In the United States, how will those providers be paid or regulated? On a totally unmanaged, claims-based, fee-for-service basis, like Canadian primary care? If that happens, Katy, bar the door—the purveyors of technology and procedure-based care in this country will accumulate wealth beyond their fondest dreams.

Will we attempt to overcome the fee-for-service revenue opportunities by imposing detailed rules on the use of high-tech care? That brings us back to needing the wisdom of Solomon. How would we create a national health care policy on prostate cancer treatment, for example? Who would make the rule? How often would it be updated? Who would enforce it? On whom?

In other words, the Canadian system works, in large part, because the actual infrastructure of care in Canada is now fully melded into the payment structure for specialty and high-tech care. We would have to go through a massive reorganization of a much larger, more complex, more expensive, and probably highly resistant industry of specialty, hospital, and high-tech providers to get where the Canadians are now, and then the cost benefits would be highly uncertain, given where we started and the price we would have to pay to restructure.

It isn't coincidental, by the way, that many U.S. doctors, weary of the accountability for containing costs and the pressures to deliver more consistent care that are increasingly imposed on them by U.S.-managed care systems, are now suggesting that a Canadian-style single-payer system might be preferable. For U.S. specialty doctors, importing only the administrative features of a Canadian fee-for-service, single-payer billing system—with no budgets, no prepayment, and no questions asked about the volumes or legitimacy of care—is a throwback to the golden age of fee-for-service medicine. Many U.S. doctors and hospitals want that fee-for-service single-payer system for exactly the same reasons we can't afford to give it to them.

Administrative Cost Efficiency/Inefficiency

One final point. To the extent that the Canadian single-payer approach looks attractive due to its low administrative costs (11 percent of total costs, as compared to an average of 24 percent in the United States),[1] it is important to keep in mind that the large, vertically integrated care systems in this country—like Kaiser Permanente, Group Health of Puget Sound, and other HMOs of that model—already run at a fraction of the Canadian costs. On an "apples to apples" basis, the costs at Kaiser are only 5 percent. At Puget Sound and other staff model HMOs, the total administrative costs are often less than 7 percent. These numbers compare to 11 percent for the "efficient" Canadian-style single-payer approach.

Because of its heavy reliance on fee-for-service payments for primary care and on a hospital payment approach that involves a great many separate hospital entities, the Canadian system is actually the second least efficient administrative system in the world.

We've already said that we could save, perhaps, $100 billion a year in administrative costs by using the Canadian system. If we go the next logical step and encourage the growth of vertically integrated care systems, we can do even better. In fact, the administrative difference between the Kaiser program and the Canadian system could save this country nearly an additional $50 billion a year.

Canadians are now studying U.S.-managed care to see how our most tightly organized and appropriately motivated care approaches might benefit them. It would be ironic for us to emulate the portions of their system that they find most problematic while being politically unable to borrow the government budget control over high tech-care approaches that they find most useful.

Single-Payer Managed Competition Might Work

One approach to a single-payer model for U.S. health care that avoids both perverse fee-for-service incentives and the immense logistical difficulties of transferring this country's hospitals and medical specialists from fee-for-service payments to a budget-based revenue system has been proposed by some very progressive leaders in Washington, D.C., and state legislature arenas. Their version of single-payer national health insurance reform combines the best features of universal coverage with some key elements of managed competition by creating a single payer (the government) who purchases basic health care from competitive teams of providers and pays capitation rather than fees. That approach could force the development of care-accountable teams, who will accept capitation payments rather than a fee schedule, and could be a successful and efficient way to structure U.S. health care delivery.

The primary problem with that innovative and persuasive approach is that it will be extremely difficult—and possibly politically impossible—for the United States to move from an employer-based private health system to a government-based payment. The primary issue is how to convert current business/employer contributions to their employees' health care programs into taxes without ending up with massively increased taxes on our citizens and increased profits for the business that had been paying for health coverage.

A second but equally important challenge would be to set up competing care teams in a true market environment with minimal direct government regulation and with maximum information about health outcomes and value given to the public so that quality and efficiency can be rewarded by patients choosing the best and most effective care teams. It would be almost impossible for the government to resist regulating the competing care teams into rigidity and inflexibility—destroying the positive potential of market forces in the process.

The plan is philosophically and conceptually sound, but probably politically impossible.

PLAY OR PAY

Another health care reform proposal that has been frequently offered in this country is to require all employers to either purchase health coverage for their employees or pay a financial penalty—the "play or pay" model.

Opponents of the play or pay approach counter that its major flaw is that most uninsured small employers cannot afford the additional cost burden that would result from having either to pay the penalty or buy health coverage for their employees. That could well be, but that is the subject of another debate. The real problem with a pay or play model is that it doesn't create any health system reform on its own.

Play or pay, unaccompanied by major payment reform and health system restructuring, would simply exacerbate our current problems because its net effect would be to pump more revenue into an already bloated fee-for-service health care environment.

A play or pay approach might very commendably improve access to care for some Americans, but it would also increase the overall costs of care and would not accomplish any reform of the health care provider system. By itself as a stand-alone proposal, play or pay is clearly a nonstarter if the issue is health care costs. As part of a larger reform effort that included appropriate subsidies for less wealthy employers, however, it could be a workable piece of the solution.

UNDERWRITING REFORMS

A number of critics of the current health care system argue that we could solve most of our health system problems simply by reforming the ways that insurance companies avoid risk. In fact, reforming many insurance company practices is highly desirable public policy and ought to be done. As a stand-alone reform approach, however, it is severely flawed.

The truth is that stand-alone underwriting reform proposals carry the same access/cost trade-off as a stand-alone play or pay approach. Underwriting reform is clearly needed because it is criminal to deny coverage to so many Americans, but those of us who advocate underwriting reform also need to acknowledge that a direct and immediate impact will always be higher overall insurance premiums.

The reason for those higher premiums is simple: If insurers are required to provide health care benefits to more sick people, then the costs of insurance will go up. Paying more claims will cost more money.

That's not even economics, it's arithmetic. Since most U.S. insurance companies are, at best, marginally profitable, these additional costs cannot be absorbed by reducing their profits. The only way that insurance companies will be able to survive the increased costs will be to increase rates.

Again, like the single-payer proposal, underwriting reform cannot stand alone as the solution to our health care problems. Coupled with other health reform measures that will make care significantly more affordable, however, underwriting reform is a form of social justice, and it needs to be done.

GLOBAL BUDGETS

Yet another frequently proposed approach to care reform is the imposition—at some level—of "global budgets" or "health care revenue caps."

As you can expect from studying the highly complex, nonsystematic way we actually pay for and deliver health care in this country, that would be an extremely difficult and probably futile undertaking. Ask yourself the following questions: On whom would the caps be imposed? By what set of rules? Who would administer them?

Would we put caps on insurers' premiums but leave the caregivers alone to continue to increase their costs at will? That would quickly cause many insurers to give up the health business (not a bad outcome) and could cause others to lose money to the point of bankruptcy, even if insurers scramble to put together some sort of provider pricing arrangements to hold their costs down.

Would we impose federally determined fee schedules and mandatory care guidelines on all care providers? That would be a massive task doomed to failure for all the reasons outlined in the discussion above about the single-payer approach.

If you're still not convinced that providers in a fee-for-service environment can quickly overcome price regulations in order to achieve their desired income levels, take a look at what has happened in the past year since Medicare attempted to control the fees of specialty physicians. Since the fee restrictions were imposed, there has been a 5 percent increase in the number of procedures doctors have performed.[2]

As you might expect, the medical specialties whose fees were limited generated the highest increases in volumes of service. Radiologists—whose fees were reduced by 12 percent—increased services by 13 percent. Urologists' fees dropped 5 percent, but their volume went up 12 percent.

Coincidental? Probably not. Controls are difficult to apply successfully in a fee-for-service environment because they are so easy to bend. It's pretty clear that price controls—like underwriting reform and play or pay approaches—will not work as stand-alone reform mechanisms. It is possible, however, for provider revenue controls to have a positive result as part of a larger reform strategy.

Short-term provider revenue controls could help create some short-term savings *if* they are done as part of a transition to a carefully restructured health care delivery system whose basic payment approach is not fee-for-service. Revenue caps for both insurers and providers could be used to encourage them to move as quickly as possible to that new environment.

Why can't provider revenue caps work as a stand-alone approach in this country if they have been successful in other countries? They work there because those countries do not rely on a fee-for-service payment system for providers. Those countries use direct control of the budget in each provider setting to achieve the savings.

If the government can directly match the operating budget of its own care system to its designated health care revenue cap, the deal is pretty much done. Once the government's budget determination is made, the care providers take the approved budget and stretch it as far as they can to meet the needs of the patients they serve within the definitions they have.

That's how the hospital and specialty-care systems in Britain and Canada work, and the approach clearly saves money.

In the U.S. health care nonsystem, however, provider revenue targets and strategies are set by millions of independent profit centers. We do not have any way to establish governmentally approved budgets for each of these caregivers. If we keep that million-profit-center system in place, then we need to be honest with ourselves about the fact that revenue caps would not directly control either revenue or costs. At best, tight controls over fees for individual units of care might temporarily slow the rate of increase, although we already have ample evidence showing that approach doesn't work for more than a very brief time. The likelihood is that revenue caps and global budgets imposed on our current environment would create a monumental bureaucratic mess, and the process could fail of its own complexity.

We have already tested government-run health system global budgeting in this country in a number of areas. Medicare, Medicaid, veterans' hospitals and other U.S. military hospitals, and the Indian health services come quickly to mind. None of these programs can be considered an unqualified success.

If we do move in that direction, we may be able to learn something about a wider application by studying these examples.

BUY RIGHT

Another reform proposal that has its advocates is the purely market driven approach known as Buy Right, which contends that the major flaw in the current health care delivery nonsystem is that health care in this country does not function as a true market in the classical economic sense.

According to Dr. Walter McClure, the prime architect of the Buy Right strategy, health care can be transformed into an efficiency-generating market environment if we put in place the tools and rules of a market. McClure contends that if consumers are given sufficient information about the relative value of the care being delivered by the care providers in each community, they will tend to select the caregivers with the best outcomes and most reasonable prices. That selection process will reward those caregivers by giving them volumes of patients, and it will penalize the poorer-quality and higher-cost providers since their proven shortcomings will cause patients to avoid them.

McClure's Center for Policy Studies has done some important projects in various communities that demonstrate the differences between various caregivers. The most recent Buy Right type of study, including data for 35 hospitals and 170 cardiac surgeons in Pennsylvania, showed that hospitals vary widely in their coronary bypass mortality rates.[3] That study also showed that the costs the various hospitals charged had *no* relationship to the quality of their care outcomes.

In fact, the highest-priced hospital in the study had an average cost per case of $83,851 and an outcomes level that was significantly below the community average. The lowest-priced hospital in the study, on the other hand, showed a charge of only $21,063 per case and reported a death rate that was significantly better than community performances.

In each case, the hospital's cases were carefully reviewed for the relative severity of the patients they were treating, with the outcomes measured relative to each hospital's own patient mix.

As McClure points out, "The power of informed customers can be brought to bear to revolutionize the health care industry for quality and economy, if patients are given ample, understandable information on the health care product. . . . The key is to define quality in terms of *outcomes and patient satisfaction,* not arcane clinical services and criteria. . . . Consumers not only grasp this information quickly. Combined with appropriate incentives, they will use it to choose providers and plans who do better for less, with the same predictable powerful results on quality and efficiency as in other sound competitive industries."

The Buy Right approach has two problems that will probably not allow it, in its current form, to become the cornerstone of national health policy. The first problem is that it calls for a five-to-ten-year national implementation period. That's a reasonable amount of time for that strategy, but it is unlikely that any policymakers have the patience or the political ability at this point to wait for a ten-year solution.

The second problem with the Buy Right approach is that it focuses its attention primarily on the individual patient's choice of individual caregivers, rather than on the relative merits of competing care systems. Health care, for many reasons, will increasingly be structured as vertically integrated care systems, and consumers will choose care systems, rather than individual caregivers. Buy Right needs to be expanded to bring that dynamic into consideration.

Overall, the Buy Right strategy is brilliant and highly innovative. A great many of us who work in health care have been heavily influenced by McClure's ideas. Had the marketplace started on a Buy Right agenda ten years ago, the health cost problem in this country would be much less of an issue.

We did not have the foresight to do that, however, and now we don't have ten years.

MANAGED COMPETITION

Probably the hottest current proposal for health care reform is a series of ideas that are lumped together under the general category of managed competition. This is the basic underlying approach that was proposed to the Clinton administration by its Healthcare Task Force.

The managed competition approach believes that the best way to deliver health care is through organized care networks—or accountable health plans—that function as direct care systems and as insurers of care.

Managed competition strategists call for a marketplace in which consumers can choose between competing systems of care based on the price and objectively measured quality of care under each system.

Market reform, under current managed competition models, would be achieved primarily by creating large cooperative purchasing pools of smaller employers. These purchasing pools would, ideally, offer a number of accountable health plans to the employees of the pool members. Each employee would be able to select from various health plans based on the price, value, and measurable quality of the plans.

In each market, the health care purchasing cooperative would quickly become the dominant purchaser of care and would therefore be an excellent tool to use to achieve true health system reform.

Basically, the managed competition model is a well-thought-out approach to organizing and rewarding our health care delivery system. Leaders like Paul Ellwood, M.D., and Alain Enthoven, Ph.D., the cochairs of a progressive group of health care thinkers called the Jackson Hole Group, have developed a strong conceptual framework for health care reform in a managed competition environment. Congressional leaders like Congressman James Cooper of Tennessee and the Conservative Democratic Forum have fleshed that idea out and created legislation that is light-years ahead of any prior congressional efforts at health care reform.

Each of the managed competition proposals put forth to date contains a number of specific flaws, but they are embedded in a core of great value that deserves the chance to be proven in the field.

Three cautions should be voiced about managed competition. The first is that it will generate great opposition from a number of provider vested interests who have no desire to become accountable and also from consumer special interests who want a magical solution to health care costs that somehow preserves the current health care delivery nonsystem untouched. Those groups will raise great smoke screens to keep a managed competition agenda from being implemented.

The second caution relates to the governance of the new purchasing cooperatives. If they are consumer-led, they will probably be successful. If, however, they are run by government bureaucracies, then they will probably add less value and create unnecessary costs.

The third caution relates to the specific goals of health care reform. If the reform focuses on cost at the expense of quality, it will fail, but if it focuses on quality first, it will have a much greater chance of success.

These three points are discussed in more detail in the next chapter.

Overall, the concept of managed competition—along with the key elements of the Buy Right strategy—should be central to our national health strategy. The final chapter discusses what an overall health strategy might look like and how it could be implemented.

Chapter 8

The Solution

Health care reform in America is possible, but only if we recognize that health care is a business as well as a calling. We need to use enlightened business incentives to make care more efficient and more effective. We need to stop tinkering with old dysfunctional payment approaches and replace them with a new payment system that meets our current needs as a nation.

To make the U.S. health care delivery system work at optimum efficiency—to make the care affordable and available to all, to maximize the pursuit of quality and improved care outcomes—America must align the rewards that we create for our health care providers with our health care objectives.

That's a simple and powerful strategy.

Anyone who doubts that the performance of U.S. health care providers will change to match the financial incentives we set for them does not understand either health care providers, human nature, or basic economic reality. U.S. providers are creative and entrepreneurial. If we build such a system, they will come. If the incentives are there, they will make it work.

THE OBJECTIVES

Any health care reform effort in this country to be successful in achieving both quality and efficiency should include the following components:

1. A commitment to Continuous Quality Improvement (CQI)
2. Reward and pay caregivers as teams, not as separate businesses
3. Prepayment for provider teams, rather than fee-for-service reimbursement
4. Public reporting of health care outcomes data to consumers
5. Baseline quality standards and public health objectives for caregivers
6. Insurance industry reform
7. A truly competitive health care marketplace
8. Reorganization of rural health care
9. Universal coverage
10. Use of prepaid care systems by the U.S. government
11. Appropriate use of technology
12. Appropriate medical leadership

Each of these objectives is discussed below.

OBJECTIVE ONE: A COMMITMENT TO CONTINUOUS QUALITY IMPROVEMENT (CQI)

Estimates vary, but even the most conservative say that up to 25 percent of the health care procedures provided in this country are unnecessary. As an example, a recent study showed that out of sixty-five thousand hysterectomies performed here each year for benign cysts, the uterus was healthy and need not have been removed in forty thousand of those cases.[1]

That is not, as noted earlier in this book, an isolated example. C-sections are done in this country at a rate that is double the medically appropriate level. The overall rate of surgery done in the United States is twice as high as surgery levels for the United Kingdom and 50 percent higher than the rate of surgery in Canada. Hysterectomies, in general, are done in this country at a rate that is six times higher than Japan's and four times higher than Sweden's. Coronary bypass operations—a procedure whose net impact has been repeatedly challenged—are done in this country at a rate ten times higher than in Great Britain.[2]

From mental health to MRI testing, the list of unmeasured and basically unquestioned uses of U.S. health care resources goes on and on. We use far more of these resources more freely than anyone else in the world.

Whose Practice Is Right?

The critical question we need to answer about these differences in practice styles is, Who is right? Should the British be doing more C-sections, heart bypass surgeries, and hysterectomies? Should they have ten times as many MRIs as they do now? And use them for millions of additional patients per year? Should the Swedes be doing four times as many hysterectomies?

The answers to these questions are extremely important if we are going to create an efficient, results-oriented health care delivery system. We need to know the right number of hysterectomies, and, more important, we need to know specifically when they are called for in individual cases. We need to know if given medical procedures work and if they accomplish the goals they are targeted to accomplish. Do they measurably reduce future concerns? Do they make a significant improvement in the patient's quality of life? Do they achieve their outcomes, and what are those outcomes?

Sadly, we don't know the answers to these questions. To make U.S. health care more efficient while simultaneously improving its success and quality, we need to focus on the desired outcomes of care and we need to do a much better job of measuring and reporting our success in attaining them.

The Deming Approach—Continuous Quality Improvement

The questions raised above are most effectively answered using a process called CQI, or Continuous Quality Improvement. The concept of CQI was developed by Dr. W. Edwards Deming nearly a half century ago. Dr. Deming's basic belief is that all production—whether of goods or services—takes place as a series of processes. The results of these processes can be significantly improved if the processes themselves are clearly understood and then improved. Dr. Deming created a set of very basic—but powerful—statistical and analytical tools that enable the producer of a product or service to identify and quantify problems, analyze their relevance, and create solutions. The Deming approach focuses on the "customer" of each process and seeks to determine both what the customer's real needs are and if those needs are being met. Rather than aiming production processes at specific preset goals, Dr. Deming believed in a much more rigorous approach directed at "continuous quality improvement." A commitment to continuous quality improvement means that the outcome of a process and the process itself are under continuous review, with a formal approach used to continuously improve both process and results. This contrasts with the more traditional American management approach that focuses on specific preset goals, and whose approach to the work process can be summed up by the phrase "If it ain't broke, don't fix it."

After World War II, Dr. Deming worked with the Japanese government to help rebuild Japanese industry. By applying Dr. Deming's rigorous, data-based approach to understanding work processes and by focusing on the continuous improvement of each process in order to achieve a continuous improvement in results, the Japanese immensely improved the quality and cost of their products and became a world economic power.

Most major U.S. industries, learning from the Japanese, are now attempting to apply these same CQI technologies (or reasonable approximations thereof) to their own production processes. Some have succeeded handsomely. Others are still learning. But those same techniques have not been generally applied to U.S. health care. Most U.S. caregivers have no idea that a formal, structural quality improvement process is applicable to their practices.

Some health care providers are beginning to adapt the concepts of CQI to health care delivery, and the results are extremely encouraging. In settings where a CQI approach is used, teams of physicians and other caregivers carefully analyze both the process and results of care and develop care approaches called, variously, "care protocols," "practice parameters," "disease control processes," "medical pathways," and so on. These CQI-based care approaches tend to be up-to-date, results-oriented, scientifically valid, and consistent in the way they deal with various diseases and health conditions. Under CQI, health care providers use the best available scientific and operational data to standardize their processes and track and report the outcomes of their care.

The reaction of most consumers to the suggestion that American health care providers should follow a consistent, scientifically current, results-based approach to care is: "But I thought that's how care is delivered now. Why do we need to add CQI?"

The answer, of course, is that our health care is not delivered in any systematic way. The result of that nonsystem approach is lower quality and less efficient care than we ought to be receiving. Applying CQI approaches to care, on the other hand, does create results similar to the ones experienced by Japanese industry: *The quality of the product goes up and the price comes down.*

As one example, when uniform best-care protocols were used for the prevention of preterm births in one large clinic setting, the preterm birth rate dropped by more than 30 percent, to a number that is now nearly 50 percent below state preterm birthrate averages.[3]

Likewise, when similar uniform-care protocols were applied to the issue of repeat C-sections, the number of unnecessary repeat

C-sections was cut by two-thirds. When care protocols were applied to breast-cancer detection, the rate of early detection improved to the point where the number of cancers not detected until (potentially fatal) stage four was cut by more than 60 percent for two large clinic systems.

In each case, the quality of care improved *and* the cost of care went down when CQI approaches were applied. The preterm birth program alone saves millions of dollars annually for the patients in just that one clinic system while helping many families avoid the pain and tragedy of premature birth.

The use of consistent, scientifically based care protocols also offers another major advantage. If care-protocol development and maintenance process are done correctly, the protocols are constantly updated and doctors are kept much more current on the best available medical practices.

Keeping Providers Current

The process of keeping health care providers professionally current in this country is now—due to the splintered U.S. health care delivery nonsystem—at best a hit-or-miss process. Even the medical textbooks that doctors rely on for information when their own memory isn't sufficient are often out-of-date.[4]

According to a study done by Harvard researchers, both medical books and professional journal articles can be significantly behind the times, with delays of up to fifteen years in bringing the newest and most effective information to the medical community. The study cited instances in which as many as twenty-five thousand lives could have been saved each year in this country if the most effective practices had been included in the textbooks and followed by U.S. physicians.

Inconsistency Occurs in a Nonsystem Care Environment

Even when physicians know the best ways of delivering care, in our current care environment that knowledge isn't always used appropriately or consistently.

For example, in a recent study, 100 percent of the doctors in a large metropolitan community were given written information about the appropriate use of antibiotics for a particular surgical procedure. The information was also given to the medical directors and chiefs of surgery at every hospital doing the procedure. Then, a year later, the study reviewed all the medical records of all the patients who had received that procedure to see if the doctors had actually used the information. The results were about what you might expect of a nonsystem. Fewer than half of the doctors used the right antibiotic protocol. In fact, nearly two thirds of them chose not to follow the antibiotic protocol, and several of the patients had significant complications.[5]

Why did the doctors ignore the protocols? Because the physicians and the hospitals were not a CQI-linked team, working closely together in a structured way to standardize, monitor, and continuously improve their care processes. Everyone did his or her own thing. In some cases, the doctors simply forgot to use the antibiotics correctly and no one reminded them. In others, the hospitals injected the right antibiotic at the wrong time. In others the doctors didn't read their mail. Some doctors differed with the protocols for particular patients because protocols are *not* applicable in every case. (In those cases, the doctors may well have been right. Medical judgment is still needed when protocols are used.)

The processes involved in the application of antibiotics were inconsistent, undependable, and unmanaged. As a result they created flawed outcomes—and that is exactly what any of Dr. Deming's students would predict for a complicated set of care processes that are routinely performed in an unsystematic way.

Applying CQI to Health Care

How would a CQI-based system improve that situation?

As I noted earlier, caregivers in this country tend to be organized in separate functional units and independent profit centers, and their interaction with patients is based on incidents of service, rather than the overall health of the patient.

In a system with a CQI focus, the question asked would be, "Were the customers' real needs met by the *entire* process at hand and not just a single incident of care?"

When health care providers focus on the patient and *not* the medical technique, then the overall process of care can be noticeably changed for the better. This is not a hypothetical concept. It's real, and it's directly relevant to you as a patient. Better process creates better care.

An extensive recent study showed that when the actual results of care alternatives are statistically compiled and made available to both the doctor and the patient, the quality of the care improves and the patient's control over his or her own care decisions increases remarkably. For prostate surgery, the study showed that when the potential medical outcomes of surgical versus nonsurgical approaches were clearly understood by the doctor, and when those relative outcomes were also explained clearly and consistently to the patient, the rate of surgery *dropped* by more than 40 percent.[6]

Think about the implications of this study. When the customers of the care process—the patients—understood the real chances of success for each alternative-treatment option, they very often chose a different approach than the one the physicians had been customarily recommending.

A very important point to realize here is that until the comparative outcomes studies were done, even the urologists involved in treating these patients did not know what the real relative outcomes were for each surgical and nonsurgical alternative. When they advised patients to have the surgery, they could only rely on their own personal experience and limited data, and that data was extremely incomplete. They didn't know what percentage of patients would become incontinent or what percentage would become impotent—or even what percentage would be bothered by either of those not uncommon outcomes.

The physicians also didn't know what the long-term consequences of *not* doing the surgery were. They were trained to do surgery—not to evaluate the total spectrum of surgical and non-surgical alternatives—and their natural inclination as surgeons is to intervene surgically in care.

But when a systematic, customer-focused approach to care was applied and when the long-term impacts on the patients of each care alternative were taken into consideration, the overall care process for those patients changed for the better. Interestingly, the overall cost of care actually went down since unnecessary surgeries, hospitalizations, and complications were significantly reduced.

What's sad about that example is that it is a rarity. The U.S. health care delivery environment typically has none of that comparative information and very few care protocols, and it acts daily in myriad ways that may or may not achieve desired results or be in the patient's best interest.

Care Protocols Should Be Shared

The quality of care can be improved further by having various provider teams share the care protocols they develop and the outcomes the protocols create, so everyone can learn from everyone else.

National Clearinghouse for Protocols

We ought to create an easily accessible national clearinghouse for protocols and outcomes studies. American doctors deserve to know what works best for any given condition. They need easy access to that information. The practice of medicine is changing daily, and doctors need a more systematic way to stay current.

I had a meeting a while ago with the chief of staff of a nationally recognized hospital. When I asked him about the applicability of CQI techniques to the practice of medicine, his response was immediate: "The application of process-oriented CQI techniques to medicine will be as significant as the development of antibiotics. I'm glad that it's happening in my lifetime!"

It's clear that a major goal of the U.S. health care delivery system should be the universal use of scientifically based care protocols. The question is, How do we get doctors and other health care providers to use them? The answer is, We pay them to do it.

How can you help make this objective happen?

If you are a purchaser of health coverage, you can decide only to purchase your care and coverage from CQI-based care systems. When you and other buyers make that decision, all providers will turn to CQI approaches for care delivery. Your joint leverage as purchasers is much greater than you imagine!

If you are an individual—a consumer of health care—you can ask your employer, policymakers, legislators, and congressional representatives to support systematic and accountable care. You can also vote with your feet. If you have the choice of multiple-coverage options, ask which one has the CQI focus and the proven outcomes and select that one. If you are a government official, support health care reform that has CQI as a core belief and approach.

Only a CQI-based approach can create the kinds of care outcomes and simultaneous efficiencies we need. One of the major flaws of many managed competition reform proposals (and all regulatory reform models) is that they do not understand how important a CQI focus is to real reform. Health system reform that does not focus on continuous quality improvement as its operational cornerstone will fail.

OBJECTIVE TWO: REWARD AND PAY CAREGIVERS AS TEAMS, NOT AS UNRELATED INDIVIDUAL BUSINESSES

If we want our health care to be based on systematic and consistent application of the most current and effective medical approaches, if we want health care delivery to be efficient, and if we want our health care providers to be accountable for the cost and quality of their care, as well as for the overall health of the patients they serve, then health care providers must function as teams and not as millions of solo businesses.

Why is this true? Why can't we simply do a better job of educating, motivating, and coordinating the current nonsystems of providers?

Because health care providers working independently cannot create basic efficiencies, consistent care practices, or systems-based care-outcomes improvement and because nonsystems cannot be easily held accountable for overall quality or cost efficiency.

We can, however, hold a team of providers who work together to serve a defined population of patients accountable for the immunization rates for the population they serve. We can also hold provider teams accountable for their cancer detection rates and their cancer cure rates, and we can measure their incidence of breast surgery and their heart surgery survival rates. Teams of providers who are held accountable as a team for the costs of their care can make meaningful decisions about where and when care is delivered. They can determine most effectively which care needs expensive hospital stays, which care should be done on an outpatient basis, and which care can be delivered most appropriately in the home. As a team, they can decide where capital investments in care facilities would create the greatest paybacks in care outcomes and efficiency.

Individual providers, on the other hand, can only make their investment and care-site decisions in the context of their own revenue and profitability and may make decisions that increase their own financial gains at the expense of the overall cost and value of care.

That's sad and inefficient.

The science, cost, and practice of health care has now progressed to the point where care should be a team effort.

Traditional insurance approaches, however, do not reward or pay caregivers as teams. We pay them separately as individual-provider profit centers, and as a result these separate-provider entities have no incentive or even mechanism to create efficiency among themselves. Our fee-for-service payment system does not recognize the considerable interrelatedness of our care system, and it clearly does not recognize the need to focus on overall health goals for any given population. As a consequence, we too often focus our resources in the wrong places.

Take cancer detection. We spend too little money on early detection (such as mammography for women fifty and older), and as a result we are spending far too much money on stage four cancer treatment.

So long as the cancer specialists who treat stage four cancers are on a different team and in a different business setting from the primary-care doctors who do most cancer detection, it will be hard to make the overall system more effective. But if we create what I call prepaid, accountable care teams (PACTs) and start prepaying primary-care and specialty-care teams a fixed amount of money that includes payment for both cancer care and cures—and if we start letting the community know how well each PACT does per one thousand patients in basic areas of medical quality, like detecting cancer early and curing it once it's been detected—then we will see a whole different care system emerge, with a major emphasis on early detection and even prevention.

OBJECTIVE THREE: PREPAYMENT FOR PROVIDER TEAMS, RATHER THAN CONTINUING TO USE FEE-FOR-SERVICE PAYMENTS

In order for caregiver teams to become efficiency-focused economic teams, they need to be paid as a team. The best way of doing this is to pay them a fixed amount of money, in advance, for the care they will provide. No other single reform element is more critical than this one.

One of the best examples of the difference between prepaid care and fee-for-service care comes from the dental plan at the health system where I work. We own and operate a network of dental clinics, one of the largest in the country. We offer extremely high quality, comprehensive benefits at a very competitive price. No one in our market can offer as many benefits as we can for the price we charge, and the quality of our dental care is superb.

How do we do this?

One major reason for our success is that we seal teeth. When young people get their adult teeth, we cover those teeth with a plastic sealant before they start to decay. As a result, we reduce the number of cavities in their mouths by nearly 68 percent for a full ten years.[7]

It's a wonderful treatment. Kids avoid the trauma of cavities, drills, and fillings. We avoid the costs associated with unhealthy teeth. Everyone wins.

But that's because we are prepaid and our financial incentive is to achieve health—in this case, healthy teeth. In the fee-for-service dental world, where dentists are not rewarded for healthy teeth, it's relatively hard to find a dentist who seals teeth. If they read their professional journals, they know that it works, so why don't they do the procedure?

Three reasons come to mind. One is that sealing teeth is a laborious process. A second reason is that, although many fee-for-service insurance plans pay for tooth sealants, many others do not, and even ones that do pay for it tend to underpay with regard to the time involved.

The third reason, however, may be the most important. *When a fee-for-service dentist seals teeth, he or she is eliminating 68 percent of his or her tooth-filling business for those patients for the next ten years.* In that context, the unenthusiastic reaction of fee-for-service dentists to sealants is entirely understandable.

How many other businesspeople or organizations would actively take steps to eliminate 68 percent of their volume for a major, highly profitable product? Not many. Most would react exactly as most dentists do—they'll seal your teeth if you ask them to, but it's not a service they advertise or promote.

Check it out. Ask some dentists. Then read the dental journal articles and draw your own conclusions. Prepayment works.

When health care providers know they can increase revenue just by increasing the volume and complexity of their services, volume and complexity result. On the other hand, when health care providers know their total revenue stream is predetermined and will not be increased if they create more services—and when the providers are organized into an economic/caregiving team— then they are forced to look at ways of reducing the cost of care. One of the best ways of reducing care costs is to create health.

We need to give teams of providers a prepaid budget that they can use in creative, flexible, innovative, and effective ways to accomplish the goals of creating health and delivering care that is efficient and of the highest quality. If they can provide care for less money than the budgeted amount, the PACTs can use that money for other purposes, including reducing the premiums they charge (in order to increase their market share) or increasing their own take-home pay. If, on the other hand, the costs of care exceed the prepaid amount, the providers will have to create operational efficiencies to reduce their costs or they may find their take-home pay reduced. In a well-designed prepaid environment, the providers are rewarded for *efficiency* and their patients' good health because the financial benefits of both accrue to the providers and they are rewarded for *quality* because the number of patients who select them as caregivers will increase based on their comparative outcomes data (see Objective Four).

The concept of delivering care through closely integrated and prepaid teams of caregivers is central to the potential successful restructuring of our care system. We will not be able to bring health care costs in this country into line unless we can make some clear-eyed decisions about the actual function and structure of the care system. Prepayment creates the incentives and the tools to enable us to take that clear-eyed look.

As one example, it is increasingly evident that between 30 and 50 percent of the care now being delivered in expensive acute-care, inpatient hospitals could be delivered just as effectively and much more economically in other less costly settings. Recovery from certain surgeries or injuries, for example, can take place just as well in a skilled nursing facility at one fourth to one half the cost of providing that same care in a hospital.

The care of hopelessly terminal patients can take place more humanely and with more comfort in a hospice than in an acute-care-hospital with cost savings, again, that range from 50 to 75 percent in comparison to an acute-care hospital stay.

Up to half of the surgeries done in many acute-care hospitals could be done as well or better in an appropriately equipped outpatient surgery center, with cost savings that are, again, significant.

These kinds of efficiencies will only result from a prepaid approach to care. When the physicians on a prepaid care team have a choice between achieving system efficiencies or losing personal income, efficiency will look very attractive and will happen.

Some current health care providers could well go out of business in the process. Communities with an excess of hospital beds will probably see some hospital bed reductions. Subspecialty physicians whose quality and/or prices are not acceptable to the local care teams will need to relocate or retrain. Such events will be painful for all concerned, but they are critical if true health care reform is to occur. If we design a system that keeps all current hospitals in business at their present size (whether or not they are either efficient or needed) and if we try to keep all subspecialists supplied with patients (whether or not the surgeries they do to keep busy adds value to the patients they treat), then we will continue to have an excessively expensive system that we cannot afford.

Prepayment Can Be Badly Done

Many people fear that prepayment encourages providers to avoid expenses by skimping on necessary care and improvements.

That is a legitimate issue to raise. It can happen. In my early HMO days back in the mid-1970s, when my health plan used to prepay each primary-care doctor individually on a monthly basis, I had a woman call me up to say that her doctor in our plan had just informed her that she needed minor surgery. He also informed her that the surgery was worth $250 and the capitation payment he received for treating her was $25 per month, so she would have to wait ten months to get the care.

We, of course, called the doctor to let him know that wasn't the way the system worked, and she received her surgery.

Those early experiments in prepayment were extremely valuable because they taught the industry what worked and what didn't. Clearly, a prepayment approach that put an individual doctor at full risk for the total cost of care for his or her patients is a bad idea, both medically and actuarially. Full-risk transfer to small clinics also didn't work because the small clinics didn't have the financial backing to withstand a major, catastrophic illness for one of their patients and because care decisions that were made in the face of that level of financial pressure for the doctors sometimes were not in the best interest of the patients.

Capitation Has Significantly Improved

The good news is that over the past two decades, the science of prepayment has advanced considerably to the point where prepayment now can be used to align incentives without creating perverse consequences or unnecessary risk. Prepayment, in a modern context, means the prepayment of teams of doctors, hospitals, and other providers as a team so that the entire team has the incentive and the financial leverage to make appropriate, cost-effective, quality-based decisions about the way it provides care.

The key to consumer-friendly payment is to (1) prepay teams of providers in a way that forces them to function as systems; (2) structure the provider risk arrangements in a way that uses reinsurance approaches to spread the costs of "catastrophic" cases across a wider population in order to protect individual providers from inappropriate financial pressure; and (3) measure the quality of the provider's care outcomes while establishing basic public health-based care criteria that they must meet.

Prepayment does not turn sinners into saints. People are people and incentives are incentives, under any payment system. The financial incentives of prepayment are needed to create efficiency in the care system, but those same incentives—taken too far—can result in patients being shortchanged in their care. It would be inappropriate and counterproductive to exchange the perverse financial incentives of fee-for-service insurance for an equally perverse set of prepayment incentives that would reward providers for underdelivering care. That is *not* the recommendation of this book. The key aim in moving to prepayment of provider teams is to set up a financing system that rewards both quality and efficiency simultaneously. That's why the linkages between prepayment, care teams, quality/outcomes measurements, and CQI are so critical. If we simply switched our payment approach from fee-for-service to prepayment without requiring public measurement and reporting of health care outcomes and consumer/patient satisfaction levels, the result could be prepayment scandals about insufficient care that would rival the abuses of excessive surgery, unnecessary treatments, and wasted health care resources that we now see in the fee-for-service environment.

If we decide to reform the system and pay providers as teams, it will be important to set up a payment approach within the teams that shields individual caregivers from any inappropriate financial incentives. The newer, more sophisticated capitation arrangements will help because they tend to place individual providers at a fairly low risk level.

In some settings, the entire risk is borne by the caregiver team itself and perverse financial incentives for individual caregivers are entirely eliminated.

For example, in a staff model HMO clinic system where the physicians are directly employed by the HMO, the entire network of owned clinics is at financial risk for the cost of care for the patients they serve. The actual financial risk is borne entirely at the corporate level. Not a penny of direct risk is passed on to the physicians or other caregivers. They are all salaried, and their salary review is based on the quality of care they deliver, not on the costs of their patients' care.

How then, you might ask, if you insulate the individual doctors from the adverse-cost impacts of their care decisions, does prepayment create an incentive that works toward efficiency and quality?

The process works because the entire organization is rewarded with revenue and patients if its costs are low and its quality is high. As a result, the entire organization has quality and efficiency as its goal. Well-run staff model HMOs have a direct incentive to construct the most efficient clinics, create the most efficient computer systems, and build the care process specifically around improving the health of their members. They create a provider payment system that insulates the providers from any perverse incentives.

While insulating individual providers from direct financial incentives is possible under a prepayment system, it is extremely difficult under fee-for-service. A few large clinics (such as the Mayo Clinic) have managed to uncouple physicians' incomes from the fees that their services generate; but that is, unfortunately, not the usual approach. Unlike fee-for-service systems where the practice of medicine is too often defined by billing codes, health care under a prepaid approach can be defined by what works for the patient, whether or not a fee-for-service billing code exists for any given activity.

Health education is a good example, as it is embedded in a well-run HMO clinic system, rather than offered as a separate service. Health educators work in the clinics to help people lose weight, improve fitness, recover from nagging sports injuries, stop smoking, and thrive through many other positive programs. Partly as a result of these programs, the overall costs of well-run staff model HMOs are consistently the lowest in the market. If these HMOs were paid for their care based on a normal fee-for-service schedule, nearly 10 percent of what they do wouldn't even have a billing code and they would be forced to stop doing many of the things that really need doing to make health care better and more efficient.

Are HMOs the Future?

This is not to say that the future of health care is HMOs, exactly as they now exist and operate, or even that all HMOs do a good job. For one thing, it is just as easy to mismanage an HMO as any other organization. (I know this to be true because I have done it myself on occasion.) HMOs in some cases have done wonderful jobs of creating high-quality, cost-efficient care. Other HMOs have focused too heavily on cost containment, and service and quality have been given a lower priority. There have been stories of improper care from some HMOs that rival fee-for-service stories. Very few HMOs, however, have allowed financial incentives to lead them astray, and all existing measurements seem to indicate that, overall, HMO quality of care is equal to or better than the quality of fee-for-service care, while being significantly more efficient.

HMOs, in fact, generally incorporate most of the more significant qualities that we need to reform health care delivery in this country. The new PACT environment that this book proposes builds on the best elements of what the best HMOs have accomplished. This proposal, however, *adds* the critically important elements of CQI-based care protocols (Objective One), outcomes reporting for consumers (see Objective Four), and administrative system reform (see Objective Six) to create a market environment in which financial incentives work in favor of quality and not against it.

NOT-FOR-PROFIT PACTS

In those areas of the United States where the health care costs are the lowest and the quality is the highest (Hawaii, Rochester in New York, Minnesota), at least one major market-dominant health care plan is a not-for-profit organization. This is not coincidental. Not-for-profit health plans can have a different focus and mission than for-profit plans, and the result can be that the not-for-profit plans keep the entire local market focused from both a quality and a cost perspective.

As PACTs are created, it would be good public policy to encourage the development and growth of not-for-profit, consumer/buyer-governed health plans as a market alternative to the for-profit organizations that will spring up all over the country. Encouraging consumer-governed, not-for-profit PACTs as a major market alternative also helps ensure that the quality agenda of the PACTs will stay intact.

Prepayment Is Critical

Prepayment is a critical element in the health care reform process. We need to reward quality and efficiency, not volumes of care. So long as the basic price of health care is based on fees for individual services, the resultant incentives will cripple significant reform efforts.

OBJECTIVE FOUR: REPORTING OF HEALTH CARE OUTCOMES DATA FOR CONSUMERS

A few years ago, I had a conversation with a state commissioner of health about the quality of health care in various areas of his state.

"Let me put it this way," he said. "There are some towns in this state where the hospital and medical care is so bad that if I were driving through the town and had a heart attack, I'd tie myself to the steering wheel, put my briefcase on the gas pedal, and try to make it to the next town before I died. My chances of survival would be better if I did that than if I stopped in those towns for care."

I asked him what, if anything, he intended to do about that.

"Nothing," he said. "Those towns protect their local hospital and doctors. It would be political suicide to try to fix that mess up. Besides, I know that to be true, but I can't prove it."

Today, in a few cases, we can "prove it." The Blue Cross plan in my home state has decided to use only the best cardiologists for their managed care system. One of the criteria for "best" was the mortality rate for coronary artery bypass surgery. The Blues checked to see how many of the patients treated by each cardiology center in the state died within a month of having that surgery.

The centers they selected had a patient death rate of 1.5 percent. The ones they rejected had a death rate of 5.3 percent.

If they did a good job of ensuring that the data they used was valid and comparable, that means that your chances of dying are more than three times higher with the cardiologists they rejected than with the more effective cardiologists they decided to use.

If you are contemplating having bypass surgery, you might find these differences in outcomes not just interesting but persuasive.

(Those numbers are entirely believable. The results in our managed care setting are almost identical to the outcomes from the providers that the Blues selected.)

By rewarding the better providers with patients, the Blues created a financial incentive for quality and penalized the less effective providers by depriving them of patients. The net result is that the less effective providers will either improve or go out of business, and patients will receive better, more cost-effective care.

Minnesota is not the only place where such studies have shown similar variances in care outcomes. Dr. Walter McClure demonstrated in Pittsburgh and Cleveland that the care outcomes of health care providers can vary considerably within a given community. His Buy Right approach set up a public process that allowed buyers to make decisions about providers based on health care outcomes.

His studies showed that the death rate for adult nonsurgical coronary admissions varied from a low of fifty-five deaths per one thousand admissions in one hospital to a high of one hundred and fifty-one deaths per one thousand admissions in another nearby hospital.[8] Both hospitals were seeing patients with about the same degree of severity, so the results can't be accounted for by saying that the second hospital had sicker patients.

The results were clearly based on different care processes that produced different outcomes.

Consumers Need and Deserve Comparative Data

American consumers deserve and need to know how well their care providers perform in key areas. Consumers should know mortality rates, C-section rates, cancer detection and cure rates, and the likelihood of success for various treatment options, so quality providers can be rewarded with patient volume. And consumers should receive that information in easily understood formats that let them compare one care system with another. It's not possible to measure and report every possible health care outcome for every possible disease or condition, but it is possible to measure and report key outcome data about the most significant conditions and to expect that your care providers will use similar practices in their other areas of treatment.

The comparative outcomes reporting process needs to be structured and managed very carefully so consumers will not be misled by statistically invalid data. One of the reasons that it makes sense to have providers functioning in teams is that a team of providers acting according to common protocols is likely to generate sufficient data on a given condition so that the outcomes-based information is statistically and medically valid. That same type of information reported for a single doctor would, in many cases, involve insufficient volume and could be statistically useless.

Caregivers Are Terrified of Outcomes Measurements

Many very good caregivers are terrified of outcomes measurements for exactly that reason. They are afraid that insufficient and incomplete data will be misinterpreted and used against them. That's a legitimate concern and is a major problem for the patient as well as for the caregiver since the patient doesn't want to be misled by a statistical aberration (or insufficient data, improperly presented) into either leaving a good doctor or seeking care from a bad one.

These issues can be resolved to everyone's satisfaction. A major part of that resolution is simply to measure the performance of caregivers as teams. Measuring outcomes is not easy—and it needs to be done with great skill in order to assure relevance and viability—but it needs to be done, to create a sense of value for health care purchasers and to create a focus for the care providers.

Provider Teams Will Self-police to Improve Outcomes

Measuring caregivers as teams rather than as individuals does not let the individual caregiver off the hook of accountability. In fact, just the opposite is true. When provider teams are held accountable as teams, those teams will use their own internal management approaches to assure consistency and care quality. In most cases, those internal policing approaches will be swifter, more direct, more decisive, and more effective than might ever be possible through an externally imposed approach. If the policing comes from outside the care system, massive and cumbersome processes might be required and the potential exists for individual providers to fight continuously with external regulators about the validity of their data and the legitimacy of their findings.

Within teams, however, protocols will be used and team members will review and judge each other's per-case performance. Under a market system in which the providers are rewarded as teams for good quality and penalized for bad, the team members have a strong incentive to correct any poor performance by one of their team participants.

Data Must Be Accurate and Valid

It will be critical to avoid fraud and deceit in the reporting process. Consumers need to know the *real* infant mortality rate, not a rate made good by fudging definitions or measurements.

Therefore, the gathering and reporting of this comparative health outcomes data needs to be done in a common framework with common definitions to prevent data reporting mischief, misunderstanding, and gamesmanship. It's very likely that some form of public/private oversight process should be institutionalized to ensure that the outcomes data is accurate and that it meets the needs of the consumers and caregivers.

Patients Need Proof

To make this brave new world work, consumers must be completely satisfied that the care system or PACT they select is focused on improving the quality and outcomes of their care, *not* on denying them services or rationing care. The best way to give that assurance is by proving the quality of care through appropriate outcomes reports. Americans want the best care in the world, and this process has the potential to give it to them. Team-based, CQI-focused medical care is clearly the best—and probably the only—way to accomplish this goal.

Market Rewards for Quality Are Essential

Once the comparative quality measurements exist, it will be critical for the marketplace, including the government as a buyer, to reward the good performers with reasonable prepayment premiums and with volumes of patients in order to encourage continuous improvement in care. If this doesn't happen, the market leverage for quality will quickly disappear and the pressure constantly to improve will melt away.

Again, this is simple common sense and economic reality.

If the market wants a continuously improving health care system, it has to ask for it and then buy it when it appears. The sellers will sell what the buyers actually buy.

Any health care reform that doesn't include consumer-outcomes reporting is severely flawed and does all U.S. health care consumers a great disservice.

OBJECTIVE FIVE: BASELINE QUALITY STANDARDS AND PUBLIC HEALTH OBJECTIVES FOR CAREGIVERS

Unlike other Western nations, we do not have a series of baseline health care standards for Americans that are, in any way, effectively enforced. That situation may be due, in part, to the fact that we have never had a health care delivery or financing system that could be held truly and practically accountable for those standards.

Care providers—separated as they now are into millions of independent business entities—cannot be held accountable for public health objectives, if for no other reason than that it is extremely difficult in fee-for-service medicine to determine which doctor has the primary ongoing accountability for the general health of any given patient or patient population. The doctor-patient relationship under traditional insurance is quite fluid and sporadic, and any given provider's patient population is almost indefinable.

But if U.S. health policy evolves to the point where teams of providers treat designated and definable populations of patients who have selected them as their team of care givers, *then it will finally be possible and practical to set baseline health care standards, track their implementation, and enforce them.* That would be a major breakthrough that could change the health status of large numbers of Americans for the better!

For example, under the new system of PACTs, the childhood immunization rate can easily be a standard for which the PACTs are held accountable and against which their performance could be measured and publicly reported.

Mammography rates for target populations comes quickly to mind as another area where a basic level of care could be expected. Appropriate medical care in the first trimester of a pregnancy is yet another. The list goes on and on. The advantages of having accountable care systems (rather than unaccountable individual provider business entities) are significant when it comes to improving the performance of U.S. health care in a number of areas in which we now fall short of Western world standards.

There are clearly a number of major community health areas in which a rational and uniform approach to care would be good public policy and make great medical sense, and those agendas should be pursued.

OBJECTIVE SIX: INSURANCE INDUSTRY REFORM

It has been said before, but it is worth repeating: We have roughly forty million uninsured people in this country—and an equivalent number of underinsured people in spite of the fact that we spend far more on health care insurance than any other nation in the world.

Our approach to insurance is administratively wasteful, shamefully discriminatory, and—because we are unique among Western nations in decoupling health care insurance from health care delivery—structurally flawed.

So how can we reform our health insurance system to make it less expensive, more inclusive, and appropriately linked with the delivery of care?

As a first step, we need to tie care delivery more directly to care financing. If we purchase health care coverage from caregiver teams, that will force a coupling of finance with care. That coupling will result in caregivers having an incentive—for the first time—to be cost-efficient in providing care because they will be sharing financial risk for the cost of care. And insurers in that environment will have an incentive to work directly with the care system to improve its efficiency. Bringing insurers and caregivers into a single team with a common financial objective and reward system would in itself represent major insurance reform in this country.

A second major reform that is accomplished by forcing insurers and providers to work together relates to administrative costs. As noted earlier, we spend a truly staggering amount of money in this country on insurance-related health care administration. These costs could be reduced sharply by a closer integration of insurance and care that results in less paperwork and a more streamlined payment process. As an example, the most tightly organized care systems in this country—the staff and group model HMOs—already achieve administrative cost levels that run far below those of the praised Canadian system. A large part of the administrative cost battle will be won simply by making the linkages between care and financing more extensive.

That integration of care and service will not in itself cure all our administrative cost problems, however. At least two more reforms are need to make our insurance process more affordable.

Complex Administration

One of the major administrative burdens in our health care financing system is the multiplicity of forms and paperwork required by our thousands of insurers, HMOs, TPAs, and other payers. Every care provider has to maintain an expensive staff of people to figure out and then fill in all the forms. Then the providers have to figure out where to send the claims and how to interpret the responses.

The insurers, at the same time, receive a great number of claims with information missing, data in the wrong position, inappropriate codes, and so on, and they incur considerable expense in having to communicate by phone and letter with the caregivers to correct the mistakes.

A far simpler approach would be to create standardized claims forms for use by all carriers and regional central claims-gathering services. Providers in any given region could just send all their claims to that regional claims-distribution center, rather than to hundreds of different insurance offices. The center could use a computer to check the claims for completeness, sort them electronically, and distribute them electronically to the appropriate insurer or health plan.

The result of that simple reform would be to cut billions of dollars from U.S. health care administrative costs, with the savings occurring in the provider offices and in the insurance companies.

One of the two major administrative cost advantages of the Canadian single-payer system is that all providers in Canada use a single claim form. There's no reason that we can't do the same thing here—only more efficiently.

Small-Group Administrative Burden

The other major administrative cost advantage of the Canadian system relates to the "distribution" of insurance. In Canada, there are no "sales" expenses as such for health insurance since everyone has coverage from the government.

In the United States, on the other hand, all private insurance is sold *by* someone *to* someone, and those sales costs are not slight. In fact, for the small-group and individual marketplace, the costs are almost crippling. While very large employers spend as little as 5 or 6 percent of the premium for administrative costs, very small groups spend upwards of 35 percent. For individuals buying health insurance, more than 40 percent of the premium they pay can be spent on administration.

Why?

These very high administrative costs exist because the sales process for individuals and small groups is cumbersome and inefficient. The salespeople who prospect the small-group marketplace may have to make twenty to thirty calls before they even find someone willing to look at a sales proposal. A very efficient salesperson then might make one sale for every five to ten proposals. That means roughly one sale per every one hundred sales calls, and that sale could be for a group with only three to five covered persons.

The sales-commission costs included in the premium that is charged these three to five people has to cover the sales rep's income needs, the costs of any advertising or direct mail campaigns that generated the original "leads," plus the clerical support staff for the sales effort and some overhead costs for the sales agency or department. (If the salesperson is an independent agent and not employed by the insurer, then there are additional costs for the insurance company staff who support the efforts of the independent agents.)

These costs are just the beginning. As part of the sales process, each small-group member is typically health-screened by the insurer's underwriting department. That process adds expense, and that expense can climb if the health status of any group member is challenged or if one or more members of the group have health conditions that will cause the insurer to either reject them or to issue contracts with special exclusions, amendments, or riders designed to minimize the insurers' claims expenses relative to particular conditions.

Once all members of the group have been accepted, the insurer needs to set up the billing process for the group, issue contracts and I.D. cards to its members, and set up the files necessary to develop subsequent group rates. The salesperson then typically has to meet with the group to explain the coverage and to set up a schedule for subsequent service and renewal calls.

This entire process is even more expensive for individual sales since the sales costs are charged entirely to that single contract.

As you can quickly see, this is not an efficient process. And what I have just described is a highly simplified version of what really happens.

We need to do better. If we agree, as a society, that current insurance distribution costs are too high, then we can put in place a more streamlined approach. That less expensive distribution system can be designed around regional purchasing pools (or consortiums) for smaller groups and individual purchasers of insurance. These purchasing pools could be established by law as the vehicle through which individuals and smaller groups purchase their health care coverage. They could be established by the government, or by true cooperative organizations, established by local small employers.

Purchasing Pools Can Slash Administrative Costs

All the PACTs in a given area should be made available through such a purchasing pool. When employers purchase coverage through these pools, each of their employees can select the health plan that he or she wants from a menu of choices. Ideally, information about each health plan's premiums, care outcomes, member-satisfaction ratings, and care-site locations would be made available by the purchasing pool to the employers as well as the individual consumers within the pool so they could make informed choices about their health plan based on the value and cost of care.

The underwriting rules for all the health plans participating in the regional pool can be standardized to end discrimination based on factors such as age and gender.

Government Use of Purchasing Pools

The government could strengthen that pooled buying process by also requiring that its own employees and beneficiaries receive their care from the health plans that participate in the purchasing pools. Adding that massive volume of people to these plans would assure their importance and success.

The use of this type of purchasing pool could reduce the administrative cost burden for small groups and individuals by more than half—if the pools are well governed and well managed.

The pools could also give individual consumers an opportunity to reward provider efficiency and quality by selecting the best provider systems as their caregivers. The marketplace impact of their choices would be extremely important in encouraging providers to offer cost-efficient, high-quality care in a service environment that meets consumer needs.

The total administrative savings that are possible from a combination of integrated insurer/provider teams, simplified claims forms, and marketing to smaller groups and individuals through large regional purchasing pools could well approach Canadian levels. Ideally, information about each health plan's premiums, care outcomes, member satisfaction ratings, and care site locations would be made available by the purchasing pool to the individual consumers, so consumers can make informed choices about health plans based on the value and cost of care.

It would be important to require that the purchasing pools be established as the exclusive way of offering health coverage to the small and medium group market for any given geographic area—because if other health plans and insurers are allowed to use discriminatory underwriting approaches aimed at those same small groups and individuals, those "outside" plans might lure the healthiest persons out of the pool. If that happens, the rates within the pool will increase until the entire pool's rates become unaffordable.

OBJECTIVE SEVEN: A COMPETITIVE MARKETPLACE

A competitive marketplace for any product forces organizations to be responsive to the product's consumers.

I've written dozens of explanations of why competition in health care is important, and every one boils down to the basic fact: Competition forces the sellers to be aware of the wants and needs of the customer.

Noncompetitive environments allow the sellers of goods or services to become complacent, nonresponsive, uncreative, and even arrogant and lazy. That's particularly true in a service environment in which the customer has no alternative way of receiving services.

True Competition in Health Care Requires Outcomes Data

As managed competition advocates gain increasing visibility on the national scene, an increasing number of people are saying, "We've already tried a competitive approach in this country, and it has failed. It's time to close down the competitive marketplace and replace it with a highly regulated approach that will bring costs into line."

The truth is that we haven't really tried a competitive approach. What we've tried has been a highly dysfunctional private enterprise approach in which the value of the services being purchased has been unknown to the customer and the consumers have been insulated (by insurance) from the costs of the care decisions they make.

In other words, our market incentives have not held our providers accountable for either the cost or the value of their care. In a truly competitive environment, patients would know which providers improve health and which do not. In a truly competitive environment, the consumers would pay more money if they went to a less efficient provider and less money if they received care from an efficient provider.

In a truly competitive environment, consumers would be able to reward provider quality and efficiency with their business, thereby forcing all providers to focus on quality and efficiency.

It's time to try competition for the first time in this country.

I know from working in a number of organizations over the years that it is difficult to make progress in either service or efficiency in an organization that is not threatened by one or more competitors in the marketplace. I have also observed that highly threatening competition has a very focusing impact on an organization and external threats can lead to wonderful internal creativity and progress.

A competitive health care delivery environment in which consumers can make knowledgeable choices about the quality and efficiency of competing teams of caregivers will lead to competition in quality and efficiency. A health care delivery nonsystem in which costs are controlled by regulation and consumers are unable to measure either quality or reward price will lead to a bureaucratic, unresponsive health care system that focuses its creativity on regulations, not customers.

Those are the choices.

Let's choose competition.

OBJECTIVE EIGHT: REORGANIZATION OF RURAL HEALTH CARE

"But what about rural areas?" people ask. "It's easy to see how a managed competition approach might work in an urban environment where there are large populations and multiple caregiver organizations that can compete with each other. But what can be done in a small town where there's only one clinic and one hospital? Or even one doctor and no hospital? How would PACTs improve the delivery of care in those areas?"

Since most of the geography of this country is rural and a large percentage of the population live in one-hospital towns, these are important questions that need to be answered by any good health reform proposal.

It's increasingly clear that the solo-practice caregivers in these small communities need to be tied into larger, regional systems. In most of rural America, health care is delivered by solo practitioners whose quality of care is unknown and whose quality of life generally leaves a lot to be desired. As discussed in Chapter 2, these small-town solo practitioners work long days and are on call for patients who need after-hours care just about every night. They have a hard time getting backups so that they can take vacations or even have a relaxing weekend.

To make matters even more difficult, these solo doctors also have to create and manage their own business operations, filing claims with Medicare, Medicaid, and multiple insurers, as well as billing patients for care not covered by insurance, and then, afterward, serving as a collection agency for unpaid bills. It isn't at all difficult to understand why small towns have a hard time recruiting doctors into that highly stressful environment.

The good news is that rural health care practices do not need to be so isolated and unattractive. It's possible to have many of the advantages of a metro-area practice if the rural doctors practice as part of a regional care system.

The work done by the Fargo Clinic and the Dakota Clinic in Fargo, North Dakota, is a good example. Each of these large multispecialty clinics has expanded its scope and its service areas by acquiring dozens of tiny clinics in the small towns surrounding Fargo. In these small towns, the large clinics serve the population through a local doctor who is a full member/partner in the larger "mother clinic" and meets its stringent quality standards. The mother clinic provides evening call backup, collegial specialty services, vacation coverage, administration services such as billing and customer service, and fringe benefits for each of its small-town satellite clinics.

Pennsylvania's Geisinger Medical Center and Wisconsin's Marshfield Clinic have created similar models.

These regional clinic systems can function as true operational systems when it comes to allocating care resources. As systems, they are able to put specialists into the small towns on a regular and appropriate schedule, and they are able to serve local populations with nurse practitioners and nurse midwives when that type of care is most appropriate.

The net result of a regional care system model is that the small towns in rural areas get solid, consistent medical care and the larger, regional clinics have a steady and dependable stream of referrals that they can count on as they efficiently build their specialty practices and support operations to fit the needs of their region.

Such arrangements are beneficial for the care providers and the communities, and they constitute the core of a PACT. Once the local doctors and the regional clinics they affiliate with are prepaid as a team and begin reporting care outcomes, they will add even more value to the communities they serve. The regional care system model deserves transplantation elsewhere.

Even the lack of a local Fargo, Dakota, Marshfield, or Geisinger clinic in a given area doesn't mean that rural areas cannot be brought into a PACT environment. In areas where the doctors and/or hospitals are solo providers, they can still be encouraged to join regional or statewide PACTs established by a hospital system, a Blue Cross plan, an insurer, HMO, medical society, or some type of medical entrepreneur. Once a PACT environment is both mandated and rewarded by purchasers of coverage and care, there will be no shortage of players wanting to create and administer PACTs.

Competition in Monopoly Environments

Even in those areas of the country where the population density will only support one PACT, the result of creating that PACT will be a local health care system that is higher quality, more responsive and more accountable than the current approach to care in most areas.

Four factors will make those "solo-PACT" rural areas significantly more competitive and consumer-responsive than the current approach for rural health care:

1. *Health Outcomes Data.* Data for local providers and for the local PACT would be made available to the local marketplace for the first time ever. The folks in a small town would learn for the first time what their local caregiver's rates were for cancer detection, heart attack mortality, C-sections and other conditions and then would be able to compare them in a meaningful way with the outcomes achieved by other care systems elsewhere in their state and in the nation. This will introduce, for the first time, an element

of quality competitiveness and awareness into the rural health care marketplace. Once that data becomes available, rural consumers will demand quality that is at least comparable to that achieved in other rural regions and their PACT will be under direct pressure to use "best-care practices" to achieve those outcomes.

2. *Competitive Pricing Levels.* The second competitive factor that would be introduced into rural areas would be pricing. In areas where there are no geographically proximate competitors, the PACTs' revenue on a per-member basis could be capped at an overall annual percentage increase level that exactly parallels the cost trends in other areas of that state or region where multiple-PACT competition does exist. This approach would keep any local-care monopolies from being able to set prices unfairly.

3. *Tertiary Care Effectiveness and Cost.* The third area in which competition can exist and benefit rural areas is in the delivery of highly specialized care. Rural areas are usually only noncompetitive in primary care. Most rural areas are within the service markets of several secondary- and tertiary-level specialty-care providers. These specialist providers now depend on referrals from rural areas for much of their livelihood. They compete aggressively with each other for these referrals, and the competition takes the form of outreach programs, helicopter and ambulance transportation linkages, and wining and dining caregivers. If rural PACTs were created, specialists would undoubtedly also compete for the PACT referrals, but a PACT could insist that cost proposals and outcomes data be the basis of the competition. This would introduce both cost and quality as discernible and effective decision factors. Ideally, based on both cost and outcomes data, the PACTs could involve local consumers in the decision process.

4. *Improved Rural Primary-care Incentives and Reimbursement.* One extremely important and highly beneficial side effect of bringing the regional PACT concept to rural America is a potential redistribu-

tion of health care dollars from the specialists and subspecialists to local primary-care doctors. Specialists now tend to be greatly overpaid, compared to their primary-care peers. In our current fee-for-service payment system, specialty care absorbs the lion's share of all available medical dollars, leaving little to support rural primary care. When rural primary-care doctors negotiate with PACTs, however, the doctors can insist on receiving a larger portion of the premium dollars as a condition of joining the PACT. Because they will control the overall health care cash flow, the rural PACTs will be freed from the traditional inequities of fee-for-service payments and could simply elect to pay primary-care doctors more and specialists less. That approach, all by itself, would make rural areas much more attractive to well-qualified primary-care doctors.

There will be no shortage of specialists willing to participate in those rural PACTs since we already have a significant oversupply of specialists in this country.

Universal Coverage Creates a Workable Cash Flow for Rural Areas

If the government moves its entitlement programs into a prepayment system and ultimately creates mandatory universal coverage for all citizens in the context of PACTs, then the major rural area problems that now exist—uninsured patients, bad debt, inefficient government payments and excessive regulations—would also be noticeably mitigated. With universal coverage, almost all rural areas could create a sufficient "all-citizen cash flow" into a local PACT that could be managed by local health care providers to generate good provider incomes and high quality, cost-efficient care.

How Many Americans Can Benefit from Managed Competition?

Some current policy analysts have contended that managed competition cannot work in communities with fewer than one hundred eighty thousand citizens because that is the number needed to support three or more full-structure health plans set up as independent HMOs. Those writers are missing an important point: It may take one hundred eighty thousand citizens to support three full-sized staff model HMOs, but it only takes two thousand people to constitute a capitated risk pool that is big enough to support a prepaid primary-care physician and support staff.

The rural competitive model can be built around local risk-pool units of two thousand people, each allied with a larger regional system that provides both administrative and specialty care. The larger regional system (or PACT) would provide appropriate reinsurance coverage for each primary-care risk pool. This would spread the cost of very expensive cases across the broader population serviced by the entire PACT, to make sure that the financial risk borne by the local caregiver is not actuarially excessive. Using risk pools of two thousand people as the basic local population requirement, it is possible to extend the prepaid managed competition approach to almost all geographic areas across this entire country.

By that measure communities with upwards of four thousand people could support competition. A community of only twenty thousand people could easily support two good-sized competing primary-care clinics, each serving roughly ten thousand people. Even in a town of only four thousand, if two competing physicians practice there, and if each chooses to be allied with a different regional specialty program, then fairly effective competition between care systems could exist in relatively small communities.

It is true that competition in very small towns would have to forgo some of the structural efficiencies of full vertical integration (It would clearly make more sense for the smaller clinics to share a hospital, rather than for each to own its own, for example). But a reasonable and effective level of competition could still exist, and the results would be beneficial for all the reasons listed above.

OBJECTIVE NINE: UNIVERSAL COVERAGE

Universal coverage for all citizens should be a primary objective of U.S. health care reform. We are the only Western nation that has not been able to achieve that goal. The challenge we face is how to finance universal coverage for all citizens *without increasing the total amount of money we spend on health care.*

We can do it, but only if we have the political courage to move all health care delivery in this country into the context of prepaid care systems. When providers are in PACTs, their total revenue can be constrained for the first time ever since the PACTs will be prepaid on a premiums basis. In a prepaid system, they will be unable to generate additional revenue by performing unnecessary services. They will need to live within that fixed revenue, and, as a result, efficiency will suddenly become profitable and desirable. As efficiencies result, the PACTs could be required to pay a relatively small portion of their cash flow as a surcharge that could be used to fund coverage for the low-income uninsured. Done correctly, that surcharge would be less than the dollar value of the efficiencies that the PACTs will achieve. If the surcharge is applied evenly to all PACTs, then it will have little or no negative impact on a given plan's competitive positioning.

If the PACTs are even minimally cost-effective, they ought to be able to bring down the total cost of care for their members by at least 10 to 20 percent by their third or fourth year of operation, measured in comparison with what those costs would have been without the PACTs. That estimate is based on the typical difference in cost between a very well run HMO and the cost of comparable benefits delivered under today's fee-for-service insurance environment. A 5 to 10 percent surcharge ought to be more than sufficient to extend coverage to all currently uninsured Americans.

As an example of the possible savings that PACTs might achieve, according to a study by Foster Higgins, the current cost difference between Minnesota HMOs and the national averages for typical fee-for-service insurance plans is roughly $1,000 per year per employee.[9] These savings exist even though the HMOs offer significantly higher benefit levels. That $1,000 difference equals a savings of 27 percent from the national average cost per employee of $4,000 per year. Such savings could fund insurance for the uninsured and still provide a price break for other care purchasers.

In other words, the possibility of another win/win outcome exists if we first reform the system and then use part of the savings to achieve universal coverage. Given the fact that we now spend billions of dollars more as a nation on health care than any other government, there ought to be enough money flowing through the system to accomplish that goal.

OBJECTIVE TEN: USE OF PREPAID CARE SYSTEMS BY THE U.S. GOVERNMENT

For health care providers in this country, the government has been an unpredictable, unenlightened, and even dangerous business partner. Time after time, the government has sought to balance its books on the health care entitlement programs (Medicare and Medicaid) by arbitrarily freezing (or otherwise squeezing) the fees that it pays to providers to the point at which Medicaid providers now say they are typically collecting only 50 to 60 percent of their regular fee schedule from the feds. This process has created a great sense of distrust about the government on the part of care providers.

On the other hand, at the same time as the government has

been shrinking fees, overall costs of those entitlement programs continue to escalate. Providers learned long ago that the easiest way to beat a deep fee-for-service discount is by increasing the volume and complexity of care being delivered and/or billed.

The people who run Medicare and Medicaid are not blind to that problem. Over the past decade, the government has run a number of extremely successful experiments in prepayment. These experiments moved away from fee-for-service reimbursement to an age-adjusted, prepaid budget for each senior or Medicaid recipient who enrolled in a prepaid plan. These experiments showed that large numbers of people would voluntarily enroll in HMOs and that HMOs could notably reduce the costs of care, with their hospital day usage, for example, often running at 50 percent or less than Medicare's fee-for-service numbers.

The government should utilize the most efficient care systems available for Medicare and Medicaid enrollees, as well as for its own employees.

The Medicare and Medicaid administrative burden on the PACTs ought to be lighter than the rules and regulations now used with fee-for-service care because those regulations typically are of little value, create great expense, stifle creativity, and are needed less in a quality-driven PACT environment than they are in the revenue-driven fee-for-service world.

Senior Political Backlash

A political backlash from the senior citizens of this country could ensure that little or no reform occurs relative to their care. Congress has clearly demonstrated its extreme sensitivity to senior lobbying groups on issues relating to Medicare benefits. Perhaps the only reasonable, fair, and politically astute approach would be to encourage seniors to enroll in PACTs by basing their Medicare premium in any given geographic area on the costs of that area's best-run PACT. If the cost of the fee-for-service delivery system turns out to be 10 percent higher than the PACTs' cost, then

Medicare could ask seniors who elect to stay in the less efficient system to pay the difference in their Medicare premium.

That approach would not force seniors into PACTs, but it would base Medicare's costs on the efficiency of PACTs, and it would allow seniors the right to pay more to be in a less efficient system.

Prepayment Works for Long-term Care

The new environment would not only provide the framework for a more accountable acute-care system, but there is good evidence from another set of successful experiments—the "Social HMOs," or "SHMOs"—that there are cash savings and improved care quality to be achieved by tying tightly managed acute care to the long-term care system on a prepaid basis. Since long-term care is a major Medicaid cost worry, this is a significant issue.

The U.S. government spends $374 billion in taxes a year on health care coverage. It's time to use that money—as part of an overall health care reform agenda—to leverage reform.

That reform will occur faster than people think, once the federal government's policy direction is made clear.

Most providers will not wait for the final legislation to be passed before beginning to restructure into appropriate types of care systems. The shadow of the upcoming legislation will be almost as strong a catalyst as the legislation itself, once the government's policy direction is basically established.

Everyone in the care and financing industries knows that change is needed and that it will occur. They are all waiting to position themselves to be winners in the new environment. I predict that change will occur at a rate that will amaze everyone, if the new environment is properly structured.

OBJECTIVE ELEVEN: APPROPRIATE USE OF TECHNOLOGY

Internal studies at the company where I work indicate that roughly half of the increase in the cost of care over the past five years has been due to new prescription drugs, new technologies, new uses for old technologies, and related changes in the practice of medicine.

If those same percentages were applied to the nation's overall health bill, then one could say (very conservatively) that the cost of care in this country would be more than 20 percent lower than it is now if we had simply frozen the practice of medicine five years ago, allowing no new drugs, no new procedures, and no new technology to be introduced during that period.

That would have meant a savings of nearly $200 billion in U.S. health care costs.

That information, while interesting, doesn't tell us what conclusions we should reach about changes in the practice of medicine because it doesn't tell us what the actual results were of all of those changes. We don't know (because we as a society do not measure and compare such things in any rational and useful way) if any segment of the population's cancer death rate dropped, if the heart surgery survival rate improved, or if diabetics now live a higher-quality life as a result of those changes.

We do know, however, that we are experiencing a technology explosion in this country. We have more MRIs than anyone could ever have imagined. Hospitals have closets full of functional but obsolete lasers that have been replaced with more current models that cost millions of dollars and will also be obsolete long before they wear out.

If, as this book suggests, we create a more rational and quality-focused health care system by encouraging providers to gather into vertically integrated care teams—each competing with other care teams based on their cost efficiency and proven and publicly known quality of care—then those care teams will have a strong incentive to make rational, value-based decisions about their use of drugs and technology. The decision to purchase an MRI would (and should) be medically driven and focused on the impact that the machine might have on improving measurable care outcomes, rather than on generating additional volumes of use and revenue for consumers.

There are several issues that need to be addressed in considering new technology:

First, Does It Work?

Our goal as a nation should be to examine each new drug or technology carefully to see if it works and how it works. While that sounds like a self-evident goal, it currently isn't happening in any systematic way.

Once the technology or drug has been proven to work, the results of its tests should be made available to all doctors on an objective, scientifically valid basis, rather than having them learn about the technology or drug solely through the marketing and sales efforts of a drug company or technology manufacturer.

Second, What Does It Cost?

At the same time that the medical results of a drug or piece of technology becomes available, we need to study the cost differences between the new treatment and its alternatives and predecessors. Currently, that information isn't readily available.

Third, How Much Do We Need?

For very high-cost technology and for very rare and highly expensive procedures, it doesn't make much sense to have a significant surplus available in any given community or region. The availability of the technology ought to be "sized to fit" the needs of the region to avoid waste and redundancy.

In the context of accountable care systems, this can be done without creating excessive bureaucracy or a cost-controlling monopoly of the service.

When a new technology emerges that is very expensive and of limited or infrequent use, there ought to be a bidding process set up in each region. The buyers should be the PACTs and the government, working as a team. The sellers ought to be appropriate providers and provider systems, competing for the business.

The purchasing team should evaluate the scientific evidence about the technology, estimate the amount of technology that would be needed to meet the needs of the region for a reasonable time period, and then request bids.

Local vendors—such as university medical schools, multispecialty clinics, and hospital systems—could then offer their bids and proposals to the purchasing pool of PACTs and the government, and the purchasing pool could make its decisions.

That particular process ties new technology directly to care-systems results, prevents a redundant proliferation of any given technology based purely on its ability to generate profits, creates intelligent, scientifically based specifications for its use, and, due to the bid process, keeps prices at a reasonable level.

A key to making this process work will be a careful screening and evaluation that will identify the point at which a drug, procedure, or technology crosses the line from being experimental to being a "best practice." That, today, is a very gray area that, again, needs to be clarified by a formal process that examines each new approach carefully to see if it works and if it is cost-competitive. That process would also create a level playing field so that all PACTs/insurers could be required consistently to offer workable new technology and procedures only when they were proven to work.

In any case, a more rational approach to drug and technology use has the potential to cut the rate of increase in health care costs significantly. We need to end the hospital arms race that results in redundant capital investments, excessive technology, and unnecessary care by focusing on the outcomes of care.

OBJECTIVE TWELVE: MEDICAL LEADERSHIP OF HEALTH CARE

One of the tragedies of American health care has been the lack of progressive leadership by our physicians. Rather than taking an overall leadership role in the continuous improvement of the health care delivery system, too many medical professionals either ignore the problems of the system in order to concentrate on their own specific practices or focus their energies and talents on protecting the status quo.

The status quo is clearly inadequate.

Everyone in this country—except for organized medicine—acknowledges that the status quo is long overdue for an overhaul. Organized medicine has too often taken the position that all would be well if we could simply reform those darned insurance companies and restructure consumer benefits (by adding more painful levels of copayments and deductibles) so that patients themselves would "stop being so demanding and wasteful."

In other words, the official position of organized medicine has been that doctors are not, in any major way, part of the problem and that current reimbursement approaches are not only acceptable, they are desirable! That is a singularly unenlightened perspective to take, and it will not lead to meaningful health care reform.

Health care reform for the second half of the 1990s will occur with or without physician leadership, but it would be much more effective if it were largely led by enlightened physicians, who could bring to bear more detailed knowledge of health care process and issues than those of us who are nonphysician reformers.

I have been privileged to work with enlightened medical leadership. The intellectual leverage they can bring to bear on the care system is truly impressive. Our problem as a nation is that we have too few of these leaders. We need to embark on a crash program to train more, with a curriculum comprised of equal parts Deming, political science, and organizational development.

The problems of care-delivery inefficiency and inconsistency can only be solved by doctors leading doctors to a better, more efficient, more consistent, and higher quality care environment. If doctors work together to create a system of continuously improving efficiency and higher quality care, we will all benefit immensely. If, however, we continue with current practices in organized medicine, arguing, for example, that outcomes studies are unfair and should not be done or used, then the likelihood of medically led reform is not very high and overall reform will be less effective.

The final key to health care reform is enlightened medical leadership. We need to create it and support it.

In Conclusion

The message that I wanted to communicate in writing this book is this: Our current system does exactly what we pay it to do. We reward providers for volume and complexity and underpay them for efficiency and quality, so we have an extremely expensive and complex care system.

Our insurers are rewarded for their ability to avoid risk, and so they do. They add little or no value to the quality of care, and they spend far too much money in the selling and administration of their product.

The combined result of fee-for-service medicine and risk-adverse insurers is a wasteful and inefficient approach to care and financing that consumes more health care money than any other system in the world while leaving millions of people without coverage or care.

The villains of this book are the incentives we've created for our caregivers and insurers.

To reform U.S. health care, we need to reform the incentives we've created for both insurers and care providers. If we change the incentives and apply them equally to insurers and caregivers, the system will restructure itself very quickly in the direction that the incentives point.

I had lunch a while ago with the president of a large manufacturing company with a significant market share in medical technology. I asked him, "Aren't you a little worried about the direction we're trying to go with health care reform? Does this increased focus on outcomes and efficiency make you just a little nervous?"

"Not at all," he responded, without hesitation. "When the marketplace starts to reward efficiency, that's what we'll create. That's fine with us. We can do it either way."

I believe that's true.

So let's utilize that responsiveness to meet our overall objectives of a continuously improving, high-quality, and highly efficient health care delivery system. Let's create the incentives that create the outcomes we want. The issues are simple when you understand them. Let's pay for what we want. Then we'll get it.

Glossary

ADMINISTRATIVE SERVICES ONLY (ASO). A service in which a third party provides administrative services to an employer group and in which the employer is at risk for the cost of health care services provided. A common arrangement with *self-funded* health care programs.

ADVERSE SELECTION. The problem of attracting members who are sicker than the general population to a health plan or insurance coverage. Specifically the problem occurs when the persons who purchase coverage are sicker or higher users of care than was anticipated when the health plan or insurer developed its budget and premiums for medical costs.

AMBULATORY CARE. Health care services that do not require hospitalization of a patient, such as those delivered at a physician's office, clinic, medical center, or outpatient facility.

AVERAGE LENGTH OF STAY (ALOS). The average number of days in the hospital for each admission (total patient days incurred divided by the number of admissions and discharges during the period).

BENEFITS. Either the amount of money payable by the insurance company to a claimant, assignee, or beneficiary under insurance coverage or the health care services that a beneficiary, member, or subscriber is eligible to receive from an HMO or health plan. HMOs usually define benefits in terms of eligible services regardless of the cost of the services. Insurers define benefits as a fixed payment tied to specific covered services.

CAPITATION. A health insurance payment mechanism in which health care providers are paid a fixed amount of money each month per insured person to cover services over a period of time; a fixed, per capita payment. In essence, a provider agrees to provide speci-

fied services to HMO or health plan members for this fixed, predetermined monthly payment for a specified length of time (usually a
year), regardless of how many times the member uses the service.
The rate can be fixed for all members, e.g., $10 per month, or it can
be adjusted for factors such as the age and sex of the members, based
on actuarial projections of medical utilization.

CASE MANAGEMENT. A process in which covered persons with
specific health care needs are identified and a plan that efficiently
utilizes health care resources is formulated and implemented to
achieve the optimum patient outcome in the most cost-effective
manner.

CLAIM. A document that is sent by either a care provider or a beneficiary to an insurer for the payment of benefits under an insurance
contract.

CLOSED ACCESS. A type of health plan in which covered persons are
required to select a primary-care physician from the plan's participating providers. The patient is required to see the selected primary-
care physician for care and referrals to other health care providers
within the plan. Typically found in a staff, group, or network model
HMO. Also called closed panel or gatekeeper model.

CODING. A mechanism for identifying and defining physicians' services on a claim form.

COINSURANCE. The percentage of the balance of covered medical
expenses that a beneficiary must pay after payment of the deductible. Coinsurance usually represents a percentage of the bill charged.
Coinsurance rates generally hover in the 10 to 20 percent range but
have gone as high as 30 percent. Coinsurance and deductibles are
most commonly found in indemnity, fee-for-service insurance and
the PPO marketplace. Coinsurance is used by many employers
when purchasing coverage for their employees on a self-insured
basis. The absence of coinsurance in the prepaid HMO arena is one
of the strong marketing appeals of HMOs.

COMMUNITY RATING. The practice of setting HMO premium
rates based on the cost experience of the entire HMO membership
rather than on the costs of a given employer group. *Community Rating
by Class (CRC)* uses the same plan-wide cost data but adjusts rates for
a given group or market segment based on age and sex categories.

COORDINATION OF BENEFITS (COB). The process governing health insurance payment when an individual has two or more health insurance policies. Involving all insurance companies, HMOs, and PPOs, this process assures that an enrollee's primary health benefits are exhausted before secondary coverage benefits begin. The savings associated with an insurer or HMO identifying enrollees who have another primary insurance policy, which usually amounts to 5 to 15 percent of revenue.

COPAYMENT. A fixed dollar amount per service that is the responsibility of the beneficiary. Copayments in HMOs for prescriptions and mental health visits are examples. These copayments tend to be modest and are devices to reduce "unnecessary" utilization.

COST SHIFTING. A situation in which a health care provider compensates for the effect of decreased revenue from one payer by increasing charges to another payer.

DAYS PER THOUSAND. A common measurement of hospital utilization in HMOs that is calculated as the total number of hospital days in a year divided by the number of thousand members of the plan. For example, 60,000 hospital days per year plus 200,000 members would equal 300 days per thousand (60,000 ÷ 200 = 300 days per 1000 per year).

DEDUCTIBLE. A set dollar amount that a person must pay before insurance coverage for medical expenses can begin. Deductibles range from $100 to $2,000, with the most common deductibles in the $300 to $1,000 range.

DIAGNOSIS-RELATED GROUPINGS (DRGs). A system of classifying patients on the basis of diagnoses for purposes of payment to hospitals. The hospital's payment depends entirely on the patient's diagnosis, and not on the number of services provided by the hospital to the patient.

EMPLOYEE RETIREMENT INCOME SECURITY ACT OF 1974 (ERISA). This federal law has a major impact on state health care reform because it exempts self-insured employers from state regulation and control. ERISA also provides for reporting and disclosure requirements for group life and health plans.

EXCLUSIVE PROVIDER ORGANIZATION (EPO). A term derived from the phrase preferred provider organization (PPO). But where a PPO generally extends coverage for nonpreferred provider services as well as preferred provider services, an EPO provides coverage *only* for contracted providers.

EXPERIENCE RATING. The practice of setting insurance or HMO premium rates based on the cost experience of a particular employer group, rather than on the costs of the entire HMO or insurer. *See* Community Rating.

EXTENDED CARE FACILITY. A nursing home or nursing center licensed to operate in accordance with all applicable state and local laws to provide twenty-four-hour nursing care. Such a facility may offer skilled, intermediate, or custodial care or any combination of these levels of care.

FEDERALLY QUALIFIED HMO. An HMO that has satisfied certain federal qualifications pertaining to organizational structure, provider contracts, health service delivery information, utilization review/quality assurance, grievance procedures, financial status, and marketing information.

FEE-FOR-SERVICE. A system of paying physicians for individual medical services rendered, as opposed to paying them by salary or capitation. This traditional method contrasts with that of prepayment, in which services are covered by a fixed payment made in advance that is independent of the number of services rendered.

FEE SCHEDULE. A list of predetermined payments for units of medical service. Each health care provider and each health care insurer can determine his or her own fee schedules in this country.

FORMULARY. A list of selected pharmaceuticals and the appropriate dosages estimated to be the most useful and cost-effective for patient care. Organizations often develop a formulary under the aegis of a physician committee. In HMOs, physicians are often required to prescribe from the formulary, unless the circumstances of a given patient clearly require a nonformulary drug.

GATEKEEPER. The primary-care health plan physician who must authorize all medical services, e.g., hospitalizations, diagnostic workups, and specialty referrals, as a condition of those services being covered by the plan. For instance, a patient is not covered for a visit to a specialist without prior approval of the primary physician.

GENERIC SUBSTITUTION. A great number of prescription drugs are available either as brand-name drugs or in less expensive generic forms without the brand name. Some care systems substitute a generic version of a branded pharmaceutical for the branded product when the latter is prescribed. Some HMOs and Medicaid programs mandate generic substitution because of the cost savings.

GROUP HEALTH ASSOCIATION OF AMERICA (GHAA). A trade association of HMOs based in Washington, D.C., and considered by many to be the voice of prepaid health care. GHAA works with the government to help shape legislation and regulation for HMOs. GHAA is now open to all HMOs that meet its membership requirements. It originally restricted its membership to group and staff model HMOs.

GROUP-MODEL HMO. An HMO that pays a medical group a negotiated, per capita rate, which the group distributes among its physicians, usually on a salaried arrangement.

HEALTH CARE FINANCING ADMINISTRATION (HCFA). The federal government agency that administers the Medicare and Medicaid programs.

HEALTH INSURANCE. Protection that provides payment of benefits for covered sickness or injury. Included under this heading are various types of insurance such as accident, disability income, medical expense, and accidental death and dismemberment.

HEALTH MAINTENANCE ORGANIZATION (HMO). In broad terms, an HMO is a form of health insurance that is also responsible for the delivery of care to its beneficiaries. An HMO provides health care services for members who prepay a premium that generally covers a comprehensive range of both inpatient and ambulatory care with limited copayments. Providers typically share the risk of the cost of care with the HMO. Traditionally, there have been four main types, or models, of HMOs, classified according to the financial and organizational arrangements between the HMO and its physicians, although most HMOs today represent a combination of two or more models.

A Staff model HMO hires its physicians individually and pays them a salary to practice in the HMO facility or clinic. Because physicians in this model and group model HMOs traditionally have had few, if any, fee-for-service patients of their own, both models are often referred to as *Closed-panel HMOs*. The physicians are subject to the policies of the HMO management. Staff model HMOs often also own facilities like hospitals and nursing homes, as part of a fully integrated care system. This is the oldest model of HMO and usually the most cost-efficient.

In a *Group model HMO,* the HMO contracts with a group of physicians and pays them a set amount per patient to provide a specified range of services. The group of physicians determines the compensation of each individual physician in the practice and often shares profits. The practice may be located in a hospital setting or a clinic. Like staff model HMOs, the medical facility usually contains a pharmacy, but, in some cases, the HMO contracts for pharmacy services. Some group model HMOs also own hospitals.

An *Independent Practice Association* (IPA) contracts with individual physicians who see HMO members as well as patients covered by other types of health insurance in their own private offices. It is the ability of IPA physicians to see both HMO and private patients in their own offices that principally differentiates an IPA from a group or staff HMO. Physicians in an IPA are paid on either a capitation or a modified fee-for-service basis. An IPA HMO may also contract with chain or independent pharmacies to dispense prescriptions to members.

A *Network model HMO* is essentially a network of group practices rather than individual physicians. Each of the contracted group practices sees HMO patients as well as fee-for-service patients in its group offices.

A *Hybrid model HMO* combines attributes of more than one of the four principal HMO models and, hence, is not classifiable in any one of the four categories.

HOSPICE. A facility or program that is engaged in providing palliative and supportive care of the terminally ill and that is licensed, certified, or otherwise authorized pursuant to the law of jurisdiction in which services are received. A hospice is a care system for dying patients.

INCURRED BUT NOT REPORTED (IBNR). The financial estimate for all health services that have taken place for a given period of time for which the HMO or insurer has not received a bill or been notified of the charges. A typical IBNR estimate would be 20 percent of the budgeted total.

INDEMNITY. Insurance benefits paid in a predetermined amount in the event of a covered loss.

INPATIENT DAYS. A measurement of health plan utilization of hospital services. A patient who has been hospitalized for five days would count as five inpatient days. This measurement is most commonly used in a ratio that reports the total number of inpatient days per 1,000 members of a health plan.

LONG-TERM CARE. Assistance and care for people with chronic disabilities. The goal of long-term care is to help people with disabilities to be as independent as possible. Long-term care is needed by a person who requires help with the activities of daily living or who suffers from cognitive impairment.

MANAGED CARE. Any system of delivering health services in which care is delivered by a specified network of parties who agree to comply with the care approaches established by a care-management process. Managed care providers may receive a capitated payment for providing all medically necessary care to its enrolled members or may be paid on a fee-for-service basis. It often involves a defined delivery system of providers with some form of contractual arrangement with the plan.

MANAGED COMPETITION. An approach to health system reform in which health plans compete to serve the needs of enrollees. Under a typical proposal, enrollees would be provided a choice of plans during an open season.

MANDATED BENEFITS. Those benefits which health plans are required by state or federal law to provide to policy holders and eligible dependents.

MEDICAID. A government health program, established by Title XIX of the Social Security Act, to provide health insurance for the poor and medically indigent. Each state administers its own program. Medicaid is funded by the state and federal governments.

MEDICARE. A federal health insurance program, established by Title XVIII of the Social Security Act, for the elderly or disabled. It is funded principally by FICA payroll deductions and somewhat by general revenues. It is administered by the Health Care Financing

Administration (HCFA), Department of Health and Human Services (DHHS), of the federal government. It has a program to enable the elderly to enroll in HMOs.

MEMBER MONTH. A measurement that records one member for each month the member is effective. For example, a member who has been with a health plan for a year would be counted as twelve member months.

OPEN ACCESS. A term describing a member's ability to self-refer for specialty care. Open-access arrangements allow a member to see a participating provider without a referral from another doctor. Also called Open panel.

OUTCOME. The consequence of a medical intervention on a patient.

OUTCOMES MEASUREMENT. A process of systematically tracking a patient's clinical treatment and responses to that treatment, including measures of mortality, morbidity, and functional status.

OUT-OF-AREA. A term describing the treatment obtained by a covered person outside the network service area.

PART A (MEDICARE). The hospital insurance program that covers the cost of hospital and related posthospital services. Eligibility is normally based on prior payment of payroll taxes. Beneficiaries are responsible for an initial deductible per spell of illness and copayments for some services.

PART B (MEDICARE). The supplementary medical insurance program that covers the cost of physicians' services, outpatient laboratory and X-ray tests, durable medical equipment, outpatient hospital care, and certain other services. Part B requires payment of a monthly premium, which covers roughly 25 percent of program costs. Beneficiaries are responsible for a deductible and coinsurance payment for most covered services.

PATIENT DAYS. *See* Inpatient Days.

PER MEMBER PER MONTH (PMPM). The calculation of costs in a health plan that clarifies the extent to which total costs for a given category change in relation to total membership. For example, total hospital costs of $2,000,000 per month divided by 200,000 members equals a $10 PMPM hospital cost.

POINT-OF-SERVICE PLAN. A hybrid model that combines features of prepaid and indemnity insurance. Enrollees decide whether to use network or nonnetwork providers at the time care is needed but are usually charged sizable copayments for selecting the latter. Variants include open-ended HMOs and triple-option plans.

PREFERRED PROVIDER ORGANIZATION (PPO). A financing arrangement in which networks or panels of providers agree to furnish services and be paid on a negotiated fee schedule. Enrollees are offered a financial incentive to use doctors on the preferred list. Typically, the enrollees must pay a deductible and copayment amount of money if they receive care from a provider who is not part of the PPO.

PRIMARY CARE. Basic or general health care traditionally provided by family practice, pediatrics, and internal medicine.

REINSURANCE. Insurance purchased from another insurance company by an HMO, insurance company, or self-funded employer to protect itself against all or part of the losses that may be incurred in the process of honoring the claims of its participating providers, policy holders, or employees and covered dependents. Also called Risk-control insurance or Stop-loss insurance.

RESOURCE-BASED RELATIVE VALUE SCALE (RBRVS). An attempt to reform fee-for-service payment to physicians and other types of providers by a classification system that measures the training and skill required to perform a given health care service. Adjusting for overhead costs, geographical differences, and services rendered, RBRVS is intended to redress Medicare's tendency to overcompensate for such services as surgery and diagnostic tests and to underpay for primary-care services that involve examining and talking with patients. The new RBRVS became effective in January 1992 and represent a small step forward in the way physicians are compensated for Medicare services. (Preliminary numbers indicate that the medical specialties have already overcompensated for RBRVS fee reductions by increasing the volume of the services delivered.)

RISK CONTROL INSURANCE. *See* Reinsurance.

SECONDARY OR "SPECIALTY" CARE. Services provided by medical specialists, such as cardiologists, urologists, and dermatologists, who generally do not have first contact with patients.

SELF-INSURED/SELF-FUNDED PLANS. Health coverage in

which the sponsoring employer or union group retains the financial risk/insurance risk for the costs of the health plan. These plans will usually contract with a third-party administrator (TPA) to handle the claims payments and other administrative activities. Insurers and HMOs sometimes serve as TPAs for self-insured employers.

SENTINEL EVENT. An adverse health event that could have been avoided through appropriate care, for example, hospitalization for uncontrolled hypertension.

SKILLED NURSING FACILITY (SNF). A facility, either freestanding or part of a hospital, that accepts patients in need of rehabilitation and care who qualify for Medicare coverage. SNFs must be certified by Medicare and meet specific qualifications, including twenty-four-hour nursing coverage and availability of physical, occupational, and speech therapies.

STOP-LOSS INSURANCE. *See* Reinsurance.

SUBSPECIALTY CARE. *See* Tertiary Care.

SURGI-CENTER. A health care facility physically separate from a hospital that provides prescheduled outpatient surgical services.

TEFRA/RISK PLANS. The Federal Tax Equity and Fiscal Responsibility Act (TEFRA) provided for the establishment of Medicare risk contracts with HMOs. Under a risk contract, an HMO is prepaid each month based upon the age/sex make-up of its Medicare enrollees. The HMO is then at total risk for all services provided. Medicare identifies a minimum benefit level, and the HMO can choose to offer additional benefits. A member premium can be changed; however, a rate justification must be submitted to the Health Care Finance Authority (HCFA) for approval.

TERTIARY CARE. Those health care services provided by highly specialized providers such as neurosurgeons, thoracic surgeons, and intensive care units. These services often require highly sophisticated technologies and facilities.

THIRD-PARTY ADMINISTRATOR (TPA). A company that processes claims payments and other financial services for self-insured plans. TPAs typically handle all phases of a health plan on a fixed fee or percentage fee, without assuming any insurance risk for the utilization or costs of the enrollees.

UNDERWRITING. In one definition, this refers to bearing the risk for something, i.e., a policy underwritten by an insurance company. In another definition, it refers to the analysis of a group or individual applicant for insurance that is done to determine rates or to determine if a group or individual will be offered coverage at all by the insurer.

UTILIZATION. The extent to which the members of a covered group use a program or obtain a particular service or category of procedures over a given period of time. Usually expressed as the number of services used per year or per one hundred or one thousand persons eligible for the service.

UTILIZATION MANAGEMENT. The process of evaluating the necessity, appropriateness, and efficiency of health care services. A review coordinator gathers information about the proposed hospitalization, service, or procedure from the patient and/or provider, then determines whether it meets established guidelines and criteria.

UTILIZATION REVIEW (UR). A formal review of patient utilization or the appropriateness of health care services on a prospective, concurrent, or retrospective basis.

VERTICAL INTEGRATION. Certain components of the health care system, e.g., hospitals, physicians, pharmacies, other providers, and/or insurance functions, combining together to provide health care services as a single entity.

WITHHOLD. The portion of the monthly capitation payment to physicians withheld by some health plans until the end of the year (or other time period) to create an incentive for efficient care. The withhold is "at risk." If the physician exceeds utilization norms, he/she does not receive it. The withhold serves as a financial incentive for lower utilization and can cover all services or be specific to hospital care, laboratory usage, or specialty referrals.

WRAPAROUND PLAN. Commonly used to refer to insurance or health plan coverage for copayments and deductibles that are not covered under a member's base plan. This is often used for Medicare.

Notes

ABBREVIATIONS

JAMA   *Journal of the American Medical Association*
NEJM   *New England Journal of Medicine*

CHAPTER 1

1. W. A. Gray, R. J. Capone, and A. S. Most, "Unsuccessful Emergency Medical Resuscitation—Are Continued Efforts in the Emergency Department Justified?" *NEJM* 325, (1991), pp. 1393–98.
2. W. McClure, *The National Buy Right Strategy: A Quality-Based Consumer Choice Plan for Universal Health Care and Coverage.* Forthcoming
3. *Socio-Economic Factbook for Surgery 1991–92* (Chicago: American College of Surgeons).
4. R. S. Stafford, "The Impact of Nonclinical Factors on Repeat Cesarean Section," *JAMA,* 265 (January 2, 1991), pp. 59–63.

CHAPTER 2

1. M. Zimmerman, "Medicare: Referring Physicians' Ownership of Laboratories and Imaging Centers," Subcommittee on Health and the Environment, Committee on Energy and Commerce, House of Representatives (Washington, D. C.: United States General Accounting Office, 1989), p. 8.
2. B. J. Hillman, C. A. Joseph, M. R. Mabry, J. H. Sunshine, S. D. Kennedy, and M. Noether, "Frequency and Costs of Diagnostic Imaging in Office Practice: A Comparison of Self-Reporting and Radiologist-Referring Physicians," *NEJM,* 323 (December 6, 1990), pp. 1604–8.

3. M. Waldholz and W. Bogdanich, "Warm Bodies: Doctor-Owned Labs Earn Lavish Profits in a Captive Market," *Wall Street Journal* (March 1, 1989), p. A1.

4. Health Market Survey (December 9, 1990), p. 7.

5. *Physician's Current Procedure Terminology Book* (Chicago: American Medical Association, 1992).

6. R. Wartzman and H. Stout, "Some Seek to Profit as White House Mulls Curbs on Health Costs," *Wall Street Journal* (May 4, 1993), p. A1.

7. D. C. Coddington, D. J. Keen, K. D. Moore, and R. L. Clarke, *The Crisis in Health Care: Costs, Choices and Strategies* (San Francisco: Jossey-Bass, 1990), pp. 8–9.

8. J. Lomas, J. C. Fooks, T. Rice, and R. J. Labelle, "Paying Physicians in Canada: Minding Our Ps and Qs," *Health Affairs* (March 1989), pp. 80–102.

9. J. J. Weiss, "Fatal Mistakes," *Ladies' Home Journal* (June 1988), p. 101.

10. W. C. Hsaio, P. Braun, D. Dunn, and E. R. Becker, "Resource-Based Relative Values: An Overview," *JAMA,* 260 (October 28, 1988), pp. 2347–53.

11. E. Weissenstein, "Hospital Executives Anxious over Ramifications of Final Physician Fee Rules," *Modern Healthcare* (November 25, 1991), p. 18.

12. L. F. McMahon, "A Critique of the Harvard Resource-Based Relative Value Scale," *American Journal of Public Health,* 80 (July 1990), pp. 793–98.

13. J. Johnsson, "RBRVS: Execs Defuse Touchy Med. Staff Issues," *Hospitals,* 65 (April 20, 1991), p. 60.

14. K. Grumbach and P. R. Lee, "How Many Physicians Can We Afford?" *JAMA,* 265 (May 8, 1991), pp. 2369–72.

15. F. L. Clare, E. Spratley, P. Schwab, and J. K. Iglehart, "Trends in Health Personnel," *Health Affairs* (Winter 1987), pp. 90–103.

16. S. A. Schroeder, "Western European Responses to Physician Oversupply," *JAMA,* 252 (July 20, 1984), pp. 373–84.

17. Grumbach and Lee, p. 2370.

18. Mary Wagner, "Demand from HMOs Raising Primary-Care Salaries," *Modern Healthcare* (August 5, 1991), p. 14.

19. A. Sager, D. Socolar, and P. Hiam, *The World's Most Expensive Hospitals* (Boston: Access and Affordability Monitoring Project, 1991), p. 1.

20. K. Oestreich, "Cesarean Sections: BCBSM Examines the Cesarean Section Dilemma," *Medical Report*, 3 (September 1989), p. 6.

21. S. A. Myers and N. Gleicher, "A Successful Program to Lower Cesarean-Section Rates," *NEJM*, 319 (December 8, 1988), pp. 1511–16.

22. R. Haynes de Regt, H. L. Minkoff, J. Feldman, and R. H. Schwartz, "Relation of Private or Clinic Care to the Cesarean Birth Rate," *NEJM*, 315 (September 4, 1986), pp. 619–24.

23. R. S. Stafford, "Cesarean Section Use and Source of Payment: An Analysis of California Hospital Discharge Abstracts," *American Journal of Public Health*, 80 (March 1990), pp. 313–15.

24. F. C. Notzen, P. J. Placek, and S. M. Taffel, "Comparisons of National Cesarean-Section Rates," *NEJM*, 316 (February 12, 1987), pp. 386–89.

25. Ibid.

26. B. L. Flamm, L. A. Newman, S. J. Thomas, D. Fallon, and M. M. Yoshida, "Vaginal Birth After Cesarean Delivery: Results of a 5-Year Multicenter Collaborative Study," *Obstetrics and Gynecology*, 76 (November 1990), pp. 750–54.

27. P. J. Placek and S. M. Taffel, "Vaginal Birth after Cesarean (VBAC) in the 1980s," *American Journal of Public Health*, 78 (May 1988), pp. 512–15.

28. R. S. Stafford, "The Impact of Nonclinical Factors on Repeat Cesarean Section," *JAMA*, 265 (January 2, 1991), pp. 59–63.

29. E. J. Quilligan, "Cesarean Section: Modern Perspectives," *Management of High-Risk Pregnancy*, 2nd ed., edited by J. Queenan (Oradell, NJ: Medical Economics Books, 1985), pp. 595–600.

30. F. P. Meehan, "Delivery Following Prior Cesarean Section: An Obstetrician's Dilemma?" *Obstetrical and Gynecological Survey*, 43 (October 1988), pp. 582–89.

31. Stafford, 1991.

32. R. S. Stafford, "Formal Strategies Needed to Curb Rising Cesarean Section Rates," News release (Chicago: American Medical Association, 1990), p. 2.

33. L. Smith, "A Cure for What Ails Medical Care," *Fortune* (July 1, 1991), p. 47.

34. D. Hemenway, A. Killen, S. B. Cashman, C. L. Parks, and W. J.

Bicknell, "Physicians' Responses to Financial Incentives: Evidence from a For-Profit Ambulatory Care Center," *NEJM,* 322 (1990), pp. 1059–63.

35. Physician Services of America, "Demand from HMOs Raising Primary-Care Salaries," *Modern Healthcare* (August 5, 1991), p. 14.

36. Interview with Judy Brown, Health·and Welfare Department, Canada, 1991.

37. Interview with John Ford, British Medical Association, Economic Research Unit, 1991.

38. American Group Practice Association, "Cardiovascular Surgeons Received Top Pay in 1990," *Modern Healthcare* (October 14, 1991), p. 10.

39. Brown interview.

40. Ford interview.

41. U. S. Congress. Congressional Research Service, "Medical Malpractice," a report prepared at the request of the House Committee on Ways and Means, Ways and Means Committee Serial 101–26 (Washington, D.C.: Government Printing Office, April 26, 1990).

42. A. R. Meyers, "Lumping It: The Hidden Denominator of the Medical Malpractice Crisis," *American Journal of Public Health,* 77 (December 1987), pp. 1544–48.

43. R. A. Reynolds, J. A. Rizzo, and M. L. Gonzalez, "The Cost of Medical Professional Liability," *JAMA,* 257 (May 22, 1987), pp. 2776–81.

44. T. A. Brennan, L. L. Leape, N. M. Laire, L. Hebert, A. A. Localio, A. G. Lawthers, J. P. Newhouse, P. C. Weiler, and H. H. Hiatt, "Incidence of Adverse Events and Negligence in Hospitalized Patients: Results of the Harvard Medical Practice Study I," *NEJM,* 324 (February 7, 1991), pp. 370–76; L. L. Leape, T. A. Brennan, N. Laird, A. G. Lawthers, A. R. Localio, B. A. Barnes, L. Hebert, J. P. Newhouse, P. C. Weiler, and H. Hiatt, "The Nature of Adverse Events in Hospitalized Patients: Results of the Harvard Medical Practice Study II," *NEJM,* 324 (February 7, 1991), pp. 377–84.

45. A. O. Berg, "Variations among Family Physicians' Management Strategies for Lower Urinary Tract Infection in Women: A Report from The Washington Family Physicians Collaborative Research Network," *Journal of the American Board of Family Practices,* (September/October 1991), pp. 327–30.

46. G. B. Shaw, *The Doctor's Dilemma: A Tragedy* (New York: Brentano's, 1961), p. v.

CHAPTER 3

1. American Hospital Association, "Renewing the U.S. Health Care System," meeting of the Section for Health Care Systems, January 25, 27, 1990 (Washington, D. C.: American Hospital Association, March 28, 1990).
2. McManis Associates' Healthcare Strategy Group, "Look to Hospital Collaborative Efforts as the Wave of the Future," *Health Care Competition Week* (October 15, 1990).
3. Ibid.
4. Louis Harris and Associates, "Trade-offs and Choices: Health Policy Options for the 1990s," *Modern HealthCare,* (February 11, 1991), p. 28.
5. Deloitte & Touche, *U.S. Hospitals and the Future of Health Care* (Boston: Deloitte & Touche, 1992) p. 21.
6. E. F. Haislmaier, "Northern Discomfort: The Ills of the Canadian Health System," *Policy Review,* 58 (September 1991), pp. 32–37.
7. J. C. Robinson, and H. S. Luft, "The Impact of Hospital Market Structure on Patient Volume, Average Length of Stay, and the Cost of Care," *Journal of Health Economics,* 4 (1985), pp. 333–56.
8. D. Mayer, "Lower Empty Hospital Bed Estimate Won't Relax Congress: Study Paints Rosier Excess-Capacity Picture, but Impact on Budget Debate Seems Slight," *HealthWeek,* 7 (May 21, 1990), p. 7.
9. S. Alnes, "MMS Had Patients, but Not Enough Who Could Pay," *Minnesota Journal,* 8 (July 9, 1991), p. 6.
10. G. Slovut, "Fifteen-City Study Finds our Medical Cost Lowest," *Star Tribune* (June 22, 1991), p. A1.
11. Ibid.
12. E. M. Robertson, "Cardiac E.R. Can Increase Admissions, Profits, Image," *Health Care Competition Week* (December 24, 1990), p. 1.

CHAPTER 4

1. J. L. Rouleau et al., "A Comparison of Management Patterns After Acute Myocardial Infarction in Canada and the United States," *NEJM,* 328 (March 18, 1993), pp. 779–84.
2. A. Swedlow, G. Johnson, N. Smithline, and A. Milstein, "Increased Costs and Rates of Use in the California Workers' Compensation

System as a Result of Self-Referral by Physicians," *NEJM,* 327 (November 19, 1992), pp. 1502–6.

3. J. M. Mitchell and J. H. Sunshine, "Consequences of Physicians' Ownership of Health Care Facilities—Joint Ventures in Radiation Therapy," *NEJM,* 327 (November 19, 1992), pp. 1497–1501.

4. B. J. Hillman et al., "Physicians' Utilization and Charges for Outpatient Diagnostic Imaging in a Medicare Population," *JAMA,* 268 (October 21, 1992), pp. 2050–54.

5. *Source Book of Health Insurance Data* (Washington, D.C.: Health Insurance Association of America, 1992), p. 52.

6. "Drug Price Hikes Limited," *Healthcare Trends Report* (December 1992), p. 5.

7. "A Prescription for Profits," *Medical Benefits* (October 30, 1991), p. 6.

8. "Drug Makers Pitch to Consumers in an Aggressive Bid for Business," *Wall Street Journal* (September 4, 1990).

9. N. W. Shammus et al., "Intravenous Thrombolytic Therapy in Myocardial Infarction: An Analytical Review," *Clinical Cardiology,* 16 (April 1993), pp. 283–92.

10. L. K. Altman, "A Costlier Heart Drug Also Proves Better," *New York Times* (May 1, 1993), p. 7.

11. M. Chase, "Genentech Drug Raises Question of a Life's Value," *Wall Street Journal* (May 3, 1993), p. B1.

12. "Prescription Drug Prices: Are We Getting Our Money's Worth?" *Medical Benefits,* 7 (March 15, 1990), p. 1.

13. "Antiarrhythmic Drug Taken Off Market," *Harvard Heart Letter,* 2 (December 1991), p. 8.

14. J. Mandelker, "Seeking the Rx for Rising Drug Costs," *Business & Health* (January 1993), pp. 24–30.

15. "Cost of Heart Revival Found to Be $150,000 a Survivor," *Wall Street Journal* (March 21, 1993), p. 15.

CHAPTER 5

1. S. Altman, "Selected Topics and Charts," presentation at Quality Management Network Seminar, Wellesley, MA, February 23, 1993.

2. *1993 National Directory of HMOs* (Washington, D.C.: Group Health Association of America), forthcoming.

3. Donald E. L. Johnson & Associates, *Marion Merrell Dow Managed Care Digest* (Kansas City, MO: Marion Merrell Dow, 1992).

4. *Source Book of Health Insurance Data* (Washington, D.C.: Health Insurance Association of America, 1992).

5. S. Woolhandler and D. U. Himmelstein, "The Deteriorating Administrative Efficiency of the U.S. Health Care System," *NEJM*, 324 (May 2, 1991), pp. 1253–58.

6. Ibid.

7. Phone communication with GHAA Legal Department, Washington, D.C., March 31, 1993.

8. Woolhandler and Himmelstein.

9. J. F. Sheils, G. J. Young, and R. J. Rubin, "O Canada: Do We Expect Too Much From Its Health System?" *Health Affairs*, 11 (March 1992), pp. 7–20.

10. Kaiser Permanente, "Environment for Innovation," Annual Report (Oakland, CA: Kaiser Permanente, 1992), p. 34.

11. G. C. Halvorson, *How to Cut Your Company's Health Care Costs* (Paramus, NJ: Prentice-Hall Information Services, 1988), p. 1.

12. Ibid., pp. 141–42.

13. Ibid., p. 121.

14. Phone communication with Todd Moller, Insurance Agents Association, Washington, D.C., March 10, 1993.

15. Halvorson, pp. 49–74.

16. Argus Health Chart, in *Findings* (Washington, D. C.: Health Insurance Association of America, April 1991), p. 3.

17. J. L. Reed and S. A. Roberts, *The Health Underwriting Cycle Revisited* (Seattle: Milliman & Robertson, 1990), p. 2.

Chapter 6

1. Congress of the United States, Congressional Budget Office, *Projections of National Health Expenditures* (Washington, D.C.: Government Printing Office, 1992), pp. 40–41; projections for 1993 were based on this data.

2. Ibid.

3. P. C. Robert, "Government Red Tape Deprives Us of Time, Earnings, Freedom," *Minneapolis Star Tribune* (July 26, 1993), p. 9.

4. *Source Book of Health Insurance Data* (Washington, D.C.: Health Insurance Association of America, 1992), p. 40.

5. Ibid.

6. *Statistical Abstract of the United States,* p. 98.

7. *Source Book of Health Insurance Data,* p. 40.

8. *Health, United States, 1991* (Hyattsville, MD: U.S. Department of Health and Human Services, May 1992), p. 283.

9. *The Universal Healthcare Almanac* (Phoenix, AZ: Silver & Cherner, Ltd., 1992); projections for 1993 were based on 1990 data in Tables 10.4 and 10.5.2.

10. Ibid.

11. Ibid., Tables 10.5.1 and 10.5.2.

12. L. Page, "Schools Weighing Response to Push for Primary Care," *American Medical News* (September 1992), p. 37.

13. Personal Communication with GHAA Legal Department, Washington, D.C., March 31, 1993.

14. A. M. Rivlin and J. M. Wiener, *Caring for the Disabled Elderly: Who Will Pay?* (Washington, D.C.: The Brookings Institution, 1988), pp. 41–42.

15. Congress of the United States, 1992.

16. Rivlin and Wiener, p. 42.

17. Ibid., p. 41.

18. G. F. Will, "Tobacco Road Led to Cancer Epidemic," *Minneapolis Star Tribune* (December 26, 1992), p. 10A.

19. Personal Communication from The Tobacco Institute, Washington, D.C., March 31, 1993; twenty-five billion packs of cigarettes sold annually.

20. B. Starfield, *Primary Care: Concept, Evaluation, and Policy* (New York: Oxford University Press, 1992), p. 228.

21. S. Okie, "Disease Outbreaks Rising as U.S. Vaccinations Drop," *Washington Post* (March 24, 1991), p. A1.

22. Personal communication with Sol Mussey, Health Care Financing Administration, March 31, 1992.

23. Health Care Financing Administration, *Office of the Actuary: 1993 Ratebook* (September 1992).

24. Ibid.

CHAPTER 7

1. S. Woolhandler and D. U. Himmelstein, "The Deteriorating Administrative Efficiency of the U.S. Health Care System," *NEJM*, 324 (May 2, 1991), pp. 1253–58.

2. R. Wartzman and H. Stout, "Some Seek to Profit as White House Mulls Curbs on Health Costs," *Wall Street Journal* (May 4, 1993) pp. A1, A8.

3. N. Harris, "Pennsylvania Scorecard Focuses on Quality," *Business & Health* (Mid-March 1993), pp. 52–54.

CHAPTER 8

1. J. C. Gambone, R. C. Reiter, and J. B. Lench, "Short-term Outcome of Incidental Hysterectomy at the Time of Adnexectomy for Benign Disease," *Journal of Women's Health*, 1 (1992), pp. 197–200.

2. K. McPherson, "International Differences in Medical Care Practices," *Health Care Financing Review* (annual supplement, 1989), pp. 9–20.

3. P. M. Mark et al, "Reduction of Preterm Birth in an HMO," *HMO Practice* (November/December 1989), pp. 199–204.

4. Lawrence K. Altman, "Textbooks Fall Behind Advances in Medicine," *New York Times* (May 7, 1991), p. C3.

5. Health Education Research Foundation Study (St. Paul, MN), forthcoming.

6. R. Winslow, "Videos, Questionnaires Aim to Expand Role of Patients in Treatment Decisions," *Wall Street Journal* (February 25, 1992), p. B1.

7. R. J. Simonsen, "Retention and Effectiveness of a Single Application of White Sealant After 10 Years," *Journal of the American Dental Association*, 115 (1987), pp. 31–36.

8. W. McClure, *The National Buy Right Strategy: A Quality-Based Consumer Choice Plan for Universal Health Care and Coverage,* forthcoming.

9. "Employers' Total Health Benefits Spending Moderated in 1992," press release, Foster Higgins, New York, NY, March 2, 1992, pp. 1–9.

ABOUT THE AUTHOR

GEORGE C. HALVORSON has worked in health care financing and delivery since 1968. During that time, he has been a senior corporate officer for a Blue Cross and Blue Shield Plan, as well as the president and chief executive officer of four health maintenance organizations, two preferred provider organizations, and two insurance companies. He is a board member and officer of two national HMO organizations, and is a trustee of the National Cooperative Business Association.

He serves on the Minnesota Health Care Commission that created what may be the most sweeping health care reform package enacted by any state in the country. He also served on the Health Care Access Commission and the Health Care Regulatory Reform Commission.

He worked for a large regional hospital network, and also as a consultant and health plan developer in Jamaica, Spain, and Great Britain.

He has published many articles on health care in various professional journals, as well as writing several book chapters and occasional guest editorials and articles for the popular press. He has published two prior books—one on drug abuse in Minnesota and the other on health care costs. The latter has been used as a textbook and is included in the training programs of two multinational insurance companies.

He is a frequent speaker on health care reform topics, and also serves as a lecturer at several colleges and universities.

HealthPartners, the company he currently serves as president and CEO, is a 600,000 member not-for-profit health plan headquartered in Minneapolis, Minnesota.

ABOUT THE TYPE

This book was set in Baskerville, a typeface which was designed by John Baskerville, an amateur printer and type founder, and cut for him by John Handy in 1750. The type became popular again when The Lanston Monotype Corporation of London revived the classic Roman face in 1923. The Mergenthaler Linotype Company in England and the United States cut a version of Baskerville in 1931, making it one of the most widely used typefaces today.